THE INSIDERS' GUIDE TO NP SCHOOL

Real Faculty Tips, Secrets, and Advice for Your RN-to-NP Journey

Dr. Molly Bradshaw O'Neal
DNP, APRN, WHNP-BC, FNP-BC

All rights reserved. No part of this publication may be reproduced, stored in a retrieval system, or transmitted in any form or by any means, including electronic, mechanical, photocopying, recording, or otherwise, without the prior written permission of the copyright owner, except in the case of brief quotations embodied in critical articles or reviews.

This book is intended to provide general guidance for nurse practitioner students, clinicians, and faculty. It is not a substitute for professional training, clinical judgment, or institutional policy. The author and publisher disclaim any liability arising from the use of the information contained in this book.

ISBN: 979-8-218-90792-1
Printed in the United States of America

For information, contact:
Dr. Molly Bradshaw O'Neal | email: drmolly@npwisdom.com

Cover design: O'Neal, M. (2025). *Wise NP Owl* (Front Cover). Canva.
Editor: Penny Dawson

For my husband, Chuck, who supports me in all things. My first legacy series gift for the next generation of Nurse Practitioner Students – you can do it!

Table of Contents

Table of Contents v

Welcome & Introduction 1

Chapter 1: Is the Nurse Practitioner Path Right for You? 3
    Understanding Your Career Options Beyond the RN Role 4
    A Deeper Dive into the NP Role 11
    Choose Your NP Specialty 12
    How Much Money Can I Expect to Make as an NP? 15
    A Day in the Life of a Primary Care Nurse Practitioner 17
    Chapter Summary 18

Chapter 2: Choosing Your NP Program 21
    Practicing with a BSN Versus Becoming an NP 22
    Goodness of Fit: Degree Pathways to Become a Nurse Practitioner 23
    Goodness of Fit: Program Formats 24
    Experience Before NP School 26
    If You Plan to Teach 27
    Selecting a Quality Program: Accreditation, Format, and Clinical Placement 29
    Applications and Interviews 31
    Can I Afford It? 32
    Chapter Summary 33

Chapter 3: Succeeding in the NP Classroom 35

Preparing Your Life for the Demands of NP School 36
Orientation Readiness 37
Review University and Departmental Policies 38
Technology Readiness 38
Academic Writing Essentials 40
Writing Support Team 42
Academic Integrity: Plagiarism and the Use of AI 43
Reviewing a Curriculum and Syllabus 45
The "3 Ps" 46
Test-Taking During Your NP Program 47
Test Anxiety 50
Capstone and Scholarly Projects 52
Chapter Summary 54

Chapter 4: How to Excel in Your NP Clinical Rotations 57

The Role of Clinicals in NP Education 58
How Placement Works: Roles and Responsibilities 59
A Word on Networking 60
Your Placement Game Plan and Timeline 62
Paid Preceptorships: When and How to Consider Them 64
Using Your Workplace as a Clinical Site 67
Protecting the Preceptor Relationship 68
Professional Communication With Faculty and Preceptors 69
Documentation You Should Keep 70
OSCEs: What to Expect and How to Prepare 72
Procedures and Skills: Build Reps Intentionally 74

Chapter Summary 75

Chapter 5: Making the Most of the Final Semester of Your Nurse Practitioner Program 77

Preparing for the Certification Exam 78

Preparing a Curriculum Vitae (CV) 82

Should I Do an NP Residency Program? 85

Lifestyle, Support System, and Financial Readiness 87

Social Media Presence 91

Avoiding Comparison 93

Graduation Celebrations 94

Chapter Summary 95

Chapter 6: Interviews, Credentialing, Contracts & More 97

Finalizing Your Certification Plan 98

Job-Seeking Strategies for Nurse Practitioners 103

Accepting an NP Role and Leaving an RN Role 107

Key Elements of an NP Contract 109

Applying for State Licensure 113

Credentialing 116

National Provider Identifier (NPI) 119

Drug Enforcement Administration (DEA) Number 120

Collaborative Agreements 121

Chapter Summary 123

Chapter 7: Thriving in Your New NP Career 127

The Transition from New Grad to Professional 128

The Power of Mentorship 129

Continuing Education and Lifelong Learning 132

Leadership Development 135

Building Professional Identity 138

Retirement and Long-Term Financial Planning 141

Chapter Summary 143

Final Thoughts 145

Appendix A: Self-Assessment: Exploring Advanced Nursing Paths
.... 146

Appendix B: NP School Interview Preparation Checklist 153

Research the Program 153

Reflect on Your "Why" 153

Know the Role 154

Practice Your Responses 154

Prepare Your Materials 154

Demonstrate Professional Presence 155

Communicate Effectively 155

Be Prepared for Key Questions 155

Follow-Up and Reflect 155

Appendix C: Can I Afford It? 157

Current Debt 157

What Will NP School Cost? 157

Income During NP School 158

Projected Income AFTER NP School 158

FINAL BUDGET 158

Appendix D: Orientation Checklist 159
    Program Expectations 159
    Technology & Course Access 159
    Communication & Support 160
    Clinical Preparation 160
    Financial & Administrative Questions 160
    Personal Organization 160

Appendix E: Study Tips for Pathophysiology, Pharmacology, and Physical Assessment 163
    Pathophysiology Study Tips 163
    Pharmacology Study Tips 164
    Physical Assessment Study Tips 166

Appendix F Clinical Toolkit 169
    Clinical Bag Essentials 169
    Capsule Wardrobe for Clinicals 170
    Meal Prep for Long Shifts 171

Appendix G Common Professional Liability Insurance Providers for Nurse Practitioners 173

References 175

Welcome & Introduction

Before we begin, let me introduce myself. My name is Dr. Molly Bradshaw O'Neal. You can call me, "Molly." It is now my 26th year in nursing and my 20th anniversary as a nurse practitioner. I am certified in Women's Health (WHNP-BC) and Family (FNP-BC). I completed my undergraduate training at Eastern Kentucky University (ADN, BSN), my master's at the University of Kentucky (MSN), and my doctorate (DNP) at Rutgers, the State University of New Jersey. I am a Navy Veteran. I have worked extensively in academia and in primary care. I work now fully time for a federally qualified health center in south central Kentucky as a nurse practitioner. I do still teach for contractors, precept students, and mentor our NP Residents. Teaching is a passion. I am a former FNP program director and DNP program director. I feel qualified to share some insights with you. Hence the name, "Insider's Guide to NP School."

If you are reading this you are likely considering NP school, enrolled in NP school, or finishing NP school. I wanted to write a consolidated book to share the answers to questions I am frequently asked. I wanted to share my faculty perspective and let you in to the secrets, pet peeves, and things that annoy faculty. I wanted to share with you, as a friend and colleague, some things I wish I had been told. I want to equip you to be incredibly successful in. your own NP journey.

It's hard to believe it, but I feel I am getting closer to the end of my career. Like anything else in life, time goes so quick. So, this is the first of a series of things I want to create in what I am calling my "Legacy Series." In the Navy we would say that I am on my Twilight Tour. Some of my comments are a little spicy. There are some faculty out there that may not want the "cat out of the bag." Still, here it is, so that you know the truth. I want to tell you to be cautious in this choice. Take your time. It is an honor to be in this position and care for the people in my practice. Make a plan to serve them to the best of your ability. If this work is not for you, it's okay. There are lots of things you can do with a nursing degree. I want to speak here to those that are committed to the NP role. Do your own homework. I hope this helps.

Chapter 1:
Is the Nurse Practitioner Path Right for You?

Before you invest time, money, and energy into graduate school, it is essential to understand what the nurse practitioner (NP) role actually involves and whether it aligns with your goals, interests, and preferred way of living life. This chapter is designed to help you make that decision with clarity and confidence.

We will begin by zooming out to examine the full range of advanced nursing pathways available beyond the RN role, including both Advanced Practice Registered Nurse (APRN) and non-APRN careers. Once the options are clear, we will focus on the NP role itself, including what NPs do, where they work, how their scope of practice is defined, and how the role compares to the physician assistant (PA). You will also get a realistic look at NP salaries across the country and a "day in the life" example from an experienced primary care NP [me] to help you visualize what typical practice looks and feels like.

This chapter concludes with an overview of NP specialty options so you can begin identifying the patient population and practice focus that best match your strengths, interests, and long-term goals.

By the end of this chapter, you will be able to:

- Describe the NP role and how it compares to other nursing career paths.

- Distinguish the NP role from the PA role.

- Identify the major differences among advanced nursing career routes.

- Evaluate whether NP-level clinical practice aligns with your long-term goals.

- Assess whether the NP pathway is the right fit for you.

- Use Appendix A: *Self-Assessment: Exploring Advanced Nursing Paths* to explore your best career match.

The goal is not to choose the most familiar or popular path, but to make an informed, intentional decision about the kind of clinician and leader you want to become.

Faculty Tip

Choosing the NP path because it is "the next logical step" is one of the biggest predictors of later regret. NPs who thrive are the ones who choose this path intentionally and with financial awareness, not automatically. Some later regret both leaving their RN role and the debt incurred for a degree ill-used.

Understanding Your Career Options Beyond the RN Role

Before you commit to NP school, it helps to step back and look at the full range of advanced nursing roles available to you. Becoming an NP is one path, but it is not the only way to elevate your nursing career. Some advanced careers fall under the APRN regulatory structure, others are graduate-level nursing roles that do not require APRN licensure, and some, like the PA, share similar clinical functions but come from a different training model altogether.

If you want help comparing these roles based on your strengths, interests, and work preferences, see Appendix A: *Self-Assessment: Exploring Advanced Nursing Paths*. This assessment is designed to help you clarify which paths may be a strong fit for you.

Understanding these differences matters because each path requires different education, offers a different level of autonomy, and leads to a different kind of day-to-day practice. The goal of this section is to help you compare them clearly so you can choose a direction that fits your goals, strengths, and long-term vision.

The Four APRN Roles (Where NP Fits In)

Advanced Practice Registered Nurses (APRNs) are graduate-prepared clinicians who provide advanced, often independent care within a defined scope of practice. The regulatory framework for APRNs in the United States is defined by the APRN Consensus Model (National Council of State Boards of Nursing [NCSBN], 2008), which establishes national standards for licensure, accreditation, certification, and education. These four elements are often referred to as LACE.

According to the Consensus Model, there are four recognized APRN roles:

APRN Role	Primary Focus	Typical Work Settings	Educational Preparation
1. Nurse Practitioner (NP)	Provides primary, acute, or specialty care, diagnoses and treats illness, prescribes medications, and manages patient care across a defined patient population.	Primary care clinics, specialty practices, hospitals, community health centers, telehealth, academia, policy roles	MSN or DNP + National NP Certification + State APRN Licensure
2. Clinical Nurse Specialist (CNS)	Improves outcomes through expert consultation, education, evidence-based practice, and systems leadership rather than maintaining an independent patient panel.	Hospitals, health systems, academic medical centers, quality improvement teams, specialty units	MSN or DNP (CNS track) + CNS Certification + State APRN Licensure

3. Certified Registered Nurse Anesthetist (CRNA)	Provides anesthesia and pain management services in surgical, trauma, obstetric, and procedural environments.	Operating rooms, surgical centers, trauma centers, labor and delivery, military, outpatient procedural settings	DNAP or DNP in Nurse Anesthesia + National Certification (NBCRNA) + State APRN Licensure
4. Certified Nurse-Midwife (CNM)	Delivers reproductive, pregnancy, birth, postpartum, and newborn care, along with general women's health services.	Birth centers, hospitals, OB/GYN practices, community clinics, home birth services	MSN or DNP in Nurse-Midwifery + National Certification (AMCB) + State APRN Licensure

All APRNs share three common requirements:

- A graduate degree, such as an MSN or DNP
- National certification in their role and population
- State licensure consistent with the Consensus Model

Only one of these four roles is the NP (Nurse Practitioner). Understanding where NPs fit within the larger APRN structure helps you make an intentional decision. If you want to diagnose, prescribe, and manage patient care, the NP role is likely the right path. If your interests are centered on anesthesia, childbirth, or system-level consulting, one of the other APRN roles may be a stronger match.

Advanced Nursing Careers That Are Not APRN Roles

Nursing careers can elevate without APRN licensure or direct patient management. Many nurses pursue graduate education and leadership roles without becoming NPs, midwives, anesthetists, or clinical nurse specialists. These paths can be just as influential, better aligned with certain strengths, and may offer greater flexibility depending on your goals.

If you enjoy teaching, leading teams, building systems, solving organizational problems, using data, or shaping policy more than diagnosing and prescribing, one of these roles may be a better fit than NP school. We are not discouraging you, just encouraging you to give this decision extensive thought.

Non-APRN Roles	Primary Focus	Typical Work Settings	Educational Preparation
Nurse Educator	Teaching, curriculum design, and clinical instruction	Nursing schools, universities, hospitals	MSN or Doctoral degree (DNP, EdD, or PhD)
Nurse Administrator/ Nurse Executive	Leadership, operations, budgeting, quality improvement	Hospitals, health systems, public health agencies, corporations	MSN, DNP, or MBA in Nursing Leadership
Informatics Nurse Specialist	Integrating technology and data into patient care systems	Hospitals, EHR vendors, research orgs, telehealth	MSN or certificate in Nursing Informatics
Public Health/ Community Health Nurse	Population health, disease prevention, community outreach	Health departments, NGOs, schools, government	BSN or MSN in Public/ Community Health
Legal Nurse Consultant	Applying nursing expertise in legal cases and litigation support	Law firms, insurance companies, government, private practice	RN license + Legal Nurse Consultant Certification

Non-APRN Roles	Primary Focus	Typical Work Settings	Educational Preparation
Forensic Nurse	Nursing practice within criminal justice systems and trauma response	Emergency departments, correctional facilities, sexual assault centers	BSN or MSN + Forensic Nursing training
Nurse Researcher	Conducting scientific studies to advance nursing practice	Universities, research centers, academic medical systems	PhD or research-focused DNP
Case Manager/Care Coordinator	Navigating patients through care transitions and services	Hospitals, insurance companies, home health	RN + CCM or MSN in Case Management
Policy and Advocacy Nurse	Influencing health legislation and systems-level change	Government agencies, nonprofits, think tanks	MSN or Doctorate in Health Policy or Systems
Nurse Entrepreneur/ Consultant	Creating independent or business-based nursing ventures	Private practice, consulting firms, startups	Varies; business training helpful

NP is just one way to advance your career. If the part you love most about nursing is teaching, leading, analyzing, problem-solving, innovating, or advocating, then an NP degree may not be the best return on investment. Believe me, this is a major investment of money and time. Choosing the right path starts with knowing the full menu of options.

Key Differences Between a Nurse Practitioner and a Physician Assistant

Because NPs and PAs often work side by side and share similar responsibilities, the two roles are frequently compared. Both diagnose, treat, prescribe, and manage patient care, but they are rooted in different professional traditions. NPs come from the nursing model, which emphasizes prevention, patient education, and whole-person care. PAs are trained in the medical model, which focuses on disease, pathology, and treatment.

One of the biggest structural differences is regulation. NPs are licensed through state Boards of Nursing. PAs are licensed through state medical boards.

Both roles were created to address gaps in the physician workforce supply, but they have evolved differently over time. NPs often work more independently, especially in states with full practice authority. PAs more commonly work in collaborative or supervisory models with physicians, particularly in specialty and surgical settings.

The table below gives you a side-by-side comparison.

Category	Nurse Practitioner (NP)	Physician Assistant (PA)
Educational Pathway	Graduate nursing program (MSN or DNP). Programs emphasize advanced clinical care, health promotion, and holistic nursing principles.	Graduate PA program (Master's degree). Programs emphasize medical diagnosis, treatment, and disease pathology based on the medical model.

Category	Nurse Practitioner (NP)	Physician Assistant (PA)
Prerequisites for Admission	Bachelor of Science in Nursing (BSN) or equivalent RN-to-MSN pathway; active RN license; minimum GPA (typically ≥3.0); clinical RN experience (1–2 years typically preferred).	Bachelor's degree (any major, though many have health science or biology backgrounds); prerequisite science courses (anatomy, physiology, chemistry, microbiology, etc.); direct patient care experience (1,000–2,000 hours commonly required).◊
Training Model	Nursing model: patient-centered, holistic, focuses on health promotion, prevention, and education.	Medical model: disease-centered, focuses on diagnosis, pathology, and treatment of medical conditions.
Program Length	MSN: 2–3 years; DNP: 3–4 years (full-time).	Master's: 2–3 years (full-time).
Clinical Hours	Typical: Minimum of 500–700 hours (MSN) and up to 1,000+ (DNP), depending on specialty and school requirements.	Typical: Average of 2,000+ supervised clinical hours across multiple medical specialties.
Certifying Bodies	AANP (American Association of Nurse Practitioners) and ANCC (American Nurses Credentialing Center); National Certification Corporation (NCC), and others depending on specialty.	NCCPA (National Commission on Certification of Physician Assistants).

Category	Nurse Practitioner (NP)	Physician Assistant (PA)
Licensure Title	Advanced Practice Registered Nurse (APRN) with state NP license and national certification. *** Varies by state.	Physician Assistant-Certified (PA-C) with state medical license and national certification.
Prescriptive Authority	Independent in full-practice states; may include Schedule II-V controlled substances.	Granted under supervising physician's license; scope varies by state.
Average Annual Salary (2024 BLS)	Approximately $134,380 nationwide (range varies by state: $108,000–$173,000).	Approximately $129,480 nationwide (range varies by state: $100,000–$160,000).

◊National Commission on Certification of Physician Assistants [NCCPA], 2024

A Deeper Dive into the NP Role

According to the American Association of Nurse Practitioners (AANP, 2025), NPs are licensed, independent advanced practice registered nurses who provide comprehensive health care across the lifespan based on population of focus. NPs assess, diagnose, treat, and manage patient conditions, order and interpret tests, prescribe medications, and develop ongoing care plans. What distinguishes the role is its nursing foundation: NPs blend clinical expertise with a focus on prevention, education, and whole-person care.

In everyday practice, being an NP means thinking critically, leading with empathy, and taking responsibility for patient outcomes while still honoring the heart of nursing. You may be asked to define this role in an interview, or even by a patient, so having a clear explanation ready matters.

What NPs do:

- Take patient histories and perform physical exams

- Order and interpret labs, imaging, and diagnostics
- Diagnose and manage acute and chronic conditions
- Prescribe medications and other therapeutic treatments
- Provide education, counseling, and preventive care

Where NPs work:

- Primary care and community health clinics
- Specialty and hospital-based practices
- Telehealth and mobile care environments
- Urgent care and emergency settings
- Academia, research, leadership, and policy roles

Once you understand what NPs do and where they work, the next question is *who* you feel called to serve.

Faculty Tip

Most students choose an NP specialty based on hearsay v actual research. Shadow other NPs and choose the specialty that matches your strength and patience for the day-to-day work. Investigate job potential in your area BEFORE you start. PLEASE don't do this if it is not your FULL INTENTION to practice as an NP. Don't take a good clinical spot and just flood the market with NPs. It's not good for you or our profession.

Choose Your NP Specialty

Choosing your NP specialty is one of the most important decisions you will make before applying to school. Each specialty defines your population focus, clinical settings, and certification pathway. It also shapes the patients you will serve and the types of care you will provide. Review these options carefully and consider which aligns best with your interests, prior experience, and long-term goals. Is there a demand for the type of NP you want to be? Where will you get a job after graduation?

Primary Care Specialties

Primary care NPs focus on prevention, wellness, and ongoing management of chronic conditions. They often develop long-term relationships with patients and work in clinics, private practices, and community health settings.

1. **Family Nurse Practitioner (FNP):** Provides comprehensive care across the lifespan, from pediatrics to geriatrics. FNPs diagnose, treat, and manage both acute and chronic conditions in outpatient and community settings. This is the most versatile and widely recognized NP role. Many choose it for the flexibility it offers.

2. **Adult-Gerontology Primary Care Nurse Practitioner (AGPCNP):** Focuses on the care of adults and older adults. This specialty is ideal for nurses who enjoy chronic disease management, preventive care, and working with aging populations.

3. **Pediatric Nurse Practitioner - Primary Care (PNP-PC):** Specializes in health promotion, illness prevention, and management of common conditions in children from infancy through young adulthood. PNP-PCs often work in clinics, schools, or pediatric practices.

4. **Women's Health Nurse Practitioner (WHNP):** Provides reproductive and gynecologic health care across the lifespan, including family planning, prenatal and postpartum visits, and management of menopausal concerns. WHNPs do not manage active labor but often collaborate closely with obstetric providers.

5. **Psychiatric-Mental Health Nurse Practitioner (PMHNP):** Offers comprehensive mental health care, including assessment, diagnosis, therapy, and medication management for patients across the lifespan. PMHNPs work in outpatient, inpatient, and telehealth settings.

Acute and Specialty Care Specialties

Acute care NPs manage complex, unstable, or critically ill patients in hospital and specialty settings. These roles require advanced assessment, diagnostic, and procedural skills, along with comfort managing high-acuity cases.

1. **Adult-Gerontology Acute Care Nurse Practitioner (AGACNP):** Provides care for acutely ill adult and geriatric patients in hospitals, ICUs, and specialty practices. This specialty is well-suited for nurses with strong critical care backgrounds.

2. **Pediatric Nurse Practitioner - Acute Care (PNP-AC):** Cares for children with acute, critical, or complex chronic conditions in hospitals and specialty units. PNP-ACs collaborate closely with pediatric intensivists and subspecialists.

3. **Neonatal Nurse Practitioner (NNP):** Provides advanced care for premature and critically ill newborns in neonatal intensive care units (NICUs). Prior NICU or neonatal experience is typically required for admission.

4. **Emergency Nurse Practitioner (ENP):** Combines family or acute care preparation with additional training in emergency medicine. ENPs work in emergency departments and urgent care settings, providing rapid assessment and stabilization.

Sub-Specializing After Certification

Once you complete an NP program and obtain certification in your population focus, you may choose to further specialize within that area. Subspecialty options include cardiology, orthopedics, pulmonology, palliative care, oncology, and many others. These areas typically require additional on-the-job training, continuing education, or postgraduate fellowships. Sub-specialization allows NPs to deepen their expertise while expanding career flexibility and earning potential. This will not occur during your initial NP training. Rather, it will occur after you are working an licensed.

How Much Money Can I Expect to Make as an NP?

Compensation is an important part of any career decision, but it should be grounded in accurate, location-specific information. NP salaries vary widely by state, specialty, experience level, and practice setting. The table below shows the most recent mean annual salaries for NPs across all 50 states and the District of Columbia, based on 2024 Bureau of Labor Statistics (BLS) data summarized by Nurse.org (2025). The intention of the table is to provide a frame of reference. I recognize there are exceptions, variance, and outliers.

In addition to base salary, most full-time NP positions include a benefits package that typically adds an estimated 20–30% in additional value through paid time off, retirement contributions, health insurance, CME or tuition reimbursement, licensure fees, and other employer-provided benefits. I will remind you of this later when talking about contract negotiations.

State	Average Annual Salary	State	Average Annual Salary
Alabama	$109,650	Montana	$131,560
Alaska	$142,340	Nebraska	$127,950
Arizona	$132,920	Nevada	$138,600
Arkansas	$116,030	New Hampshire	$133,660
California	$173,190	New Jersey	$140,470
Colorado	$126,600	New Mexico	$136,620
Connecticut	$141,140	New York	$148,410
Delaware	$130,190	North Carolina	$124,830
District of Columbia	$137,600	North Dakota	$121,200
Florida	$128,340	Ohio	$121,250
Georgia	$125,490	Oklahoma	$127,120

State	Average Annual Salary	State	Average Annual Salary
Hawaii	$135,020	Oregon	$148,030
Idaho	$131,380	Pennsylvania	$126,730
Illinois	$128,880	Rhode Island	$139,600
Indiana	$126,520	South Carolina	$113,950
Iowa	$133,020	South Dakota	$122,300
Kansas	$127,900	Tennessee	$108,180
Kentucky	$116,930	Texas	$130,930
Louisiana	$124,850	Utah	$131,680
Maine	$127,750	Vermont	$130,580
Maryland	$127,100	Virginia	$122,180
Massachusetts	$145,140	Washington	$143,620
Michigan	$127,200	West Virginia	$122,140
Minnesota	$128,120	Wisconsin	$130,490
Mississippi	$122,930	Wyoming	$126,060
Missouri	$124,600		

Nurse.org (BLS-summarized data)
Nurse.org. (2025, May 14). *Nurse practitioner salary by state (BLS 2024 OEWS data)*. https://nurse.org/resources/nurse-practitioner-salary/

Indeed (supplemental salary averages)
Indeed. (2025). *Average nurse practitioner salary*. Indeed Career Guide. https://www.indeed.com/career/nurse-practitioner/salaries

A Day in the Life of a Primary Care Nurse Practitioner

Before you commit to NP school, talk to NPs who are actually doing the work you think you want to do. Shadow them if you can. When I interview NP applicants, one of my first questions is always, "How much time have you spent observing or speaking with practicing NPs?" Vague answers almost always signal uncertain motivation.

While workload and schedules vary by region and practice setting, here is what my typical days look like after more than twenty years in primary care.

I am certified as both a Family Nurse Practitioner and a Women's Health Nurse Practitioner, and I practice in a federally qualified health center (FQHC). On a typical day, I see 26–30 patients, from newborns to older adults. I usually arrive by 7:00 a.m. to review labs, messages, and my schedule before appointments start at 8:00 a.m. The work is a mix of chronic disease management, well-woman exams, urgent complaints, prenatal visits, and preventive care.

Primary care is team-based by design I have a dedicated RN who works only with me. Another nurse helps with nurse tasks like injections, calls, EKGs, etc. In my office we have a lab tech, xray tech, and counselors. I speak regularly to pharmacists, mostly on the phone. That collaboration is one of the best parts of the job. Everyone stays in their lane, but no one works alone.

Lunch is scheduled for an hour, but I often spend part of it catching up on charting or reviewing results. There is almost always an add-on or last-minute squeeze-in. I do my best to finish documentation before leaving the office. After years of trial and error (plus some help from AI charting tools), I rarely take charts home, maybe 1-2 times per month.

My schedule is four ten-hour days each week, which gives me a three-day weekend every week. I take Wednesdays off because it is the lowest-volume day in primary care, which means I am present on the busy days that contribute more to productivity bonuses. I do not take

> calls, I do not work holidays, and I do not work weekends. That boundary is one of the main reasons I still enjoy this work.
>
> Vacations are tricky. If I am in the state/country, I sometimes check my messages in the morning. I almost never take a sick day. I limit my interactions with drug reps to one day per week to minimize distraction. I am NEVER on social media during work hours.
>
> Because I am dual-certified, I also have a strong women's health panel and occasionally make home visits for high-risk or mobility-limited patients. On the side, I teach online and do small consulting projects. That brings in an extra $40,000–$50,000 a year, but more importantly, it adds variety and keeps me connected to evidence-based practice and the next generation of NPs.
>
> This is the part of NP life people do not always talk about: sustainability. It takes time to build a schedule, a boundary system, and a clinical rhythm that you can live with long term. Once you do, primary care can offer a rare blend of purpose, stability, and flexibility.
>
> If that picture still excites you: busy days, deep relationships, broad clinical variety, and room to shape your own work-life balance, you may be on the right path.

Chapter Summary

Deciding whether to become an NP requires more than enthusiasm for "moving up" in your career. It calls for a clear understanding of what the NP role actually involves, how it compares to other APRN and non-APRN paths, and whether the day-to-day work aligns with your strengths and long-term goals. In this chapter, you explored the broader landscape of advanced nursing careers, learned where the NP fits within the four APRN roles, and compared the NP pathway to the PA route. You also reviewed common NP specialties and considered a real-world picture of life in primary care.

If you are energized by diagnosing and managing patient care, value autonomy, and want to blend clinical reasoning with a nursing-based focus on education and prevention, the NP role may be a strong fit. If you are more drawn to leadership, teaching, policy, analytics, or research, another advanced nursing role may serve you better.

Your goal is not to choose the most familiar option, but the one that matches who you are and the kind of work you want to do every day. Use Appendix A: *Self-Assessment: Exploring Advanced Nursing Paths* to begin clarifying your direction, then continue to the next chapter to learn how to choose the right degree pathway, compare programs, and prepare a competitive NP school application.

Chapter 2:
Choosing Your NP Program

Before you submit a single application, it's essential to understand the degree pathways and program structures that prepare you for advanced practice as a nurse practitioner. This chapter is designed to help you choose the educational route that best aligns with your goals, timeline, and future career plans. Is it a good fit? Is the program good quality? Can you afford it?

In regard to goodness of fit, we'll begin with a clear overview of the graduate degrees that qualify you to become an NP and what each pathway prepares you for. From there, we'll look at how to evaluate programs based on accreditation, delivery format (online, hybrid, or campus-based), and the level of clinical placement support they provide. You will also explore how your RN experience influences readiness for graduate study and how degree selection may shape opportunities for teaching or academic roles in the future.

In regard to quality of the program, there will be a section focused on applications and interviews, so you know how to present yourself as a prepared, professional candidate. Appendix B: *NP School Interview Preparation Checklist* is included so you can move directly from planning to action.

Finally, most importantly, in regard to finances, it's time to examine if you can afford NP school or not. Appendix C: *Can I Afford It?* Will help answer this question.

By the end of this chapter, you will be able to:

- Distinguish clearly between the MSN and DNP degrees.

- Examine program formats for goodness of fit.

- Evaluate a programs' quality based on accreditation, delivery format, and clinical placement expectations.

- Identify what best aligns with your current and future financial situation.

The goal should not be to finish as quickly as possible, but to choose the path that gives you the preparation, support, and confidence you need to practice safely, think critically, and grow steadily as a nurse practitioner. Financial hardships can be serious if care is not taken in the early stages of planning.

Practicing with a BSN Versus Becoming an NP

You likely know this, but just a review [in case]. A Bachelor of Science in Nursing (BSN) prepares you for professional nursing practice and gives you access to a wide range of roles in clinical care, leadership, education, community health, informatics, and other areas of nursing. Many nurses build long and meaningful careers at the bachelor's level, whether they work at the bedside, move into management, or take on roles in quality improvement, public health, or patient education.

Graduating with a BSN does not automatically make you a practicing nurse. To work as a registered nurse, you must pass the National Council Licensure Examination (NCLEX-RN) and obtain state licensure. An active RN license is required before you can apply to any NP program.

If you already have a bachelor's degree in another field (for example, psychology, biology, business, or sociology), you can still become an NP, but you must first become a registered nurse. Some schools offer "direct-entry" or "entry-level" master's programs for non-nurses. These programs allow you to complete the nursing coursework, sit for the NCLEX-RN, become licensed as an RN, and then continue into the NP portion of the degree. There is no pathway to becoming an NP that bypasses RN licensure.

Becoming an NP requires graduate-level nursing education. This happens through either a Master of Science in Nursing (MSN) or a Doctor of Nursing Practice (DNP). Both degrees qualify you to take a national NP certification exam and apply for state licensure as an NP. This advanced preparation expands your scope of practice, allowing you to diagnose, interpret tests, prescribe medications, and manage patient care as a licensed healthcare provider.

Goodness of Fit: Degree Pathways to Become a Nurse Practitioner

Once you have decided to pursue the NP role, the next choice is which educational pathway will qualify you for certification and licensure. There are two main options:

1. **Master of Science in Nursing (MSN):** An MSN program is the most common route to becoming an NP. It provides the graduate-level coursework and required clinical hours needed to sit for a national NP certification exam in your chosen specialty. After passing the exam, you can apply for state licensure and begin practicing as an NP. Many nurses choose this pathway because it takes less time to complete and is typically less expensive than a doctoral degree.

2. **Doctor of Nursing Practice (DNP):** A DNP program also prepares you for national certification and licensure, but it includes additional training in leadership, quality improvement, health systems, and evidence-based practice (American Association of Colleges of Nursing [AACN], 2021). The DNP is considered the terminal clinical degree in nursing. Some students choose to start at the doctoral level, so they only return to school once, while others earn the DNP later in their career after practicing as MSN-prepared NPs.

Both degrees prepare you to:

- Complete advanced clinical coursework
- Meet required supervised clinical hours
- Sit for a national certification exam
- Apply for licensure as an NP in your state

The difference between the two pathways is not in what you are licensed to do, but in the level of academic preparation, cost, time commitment, and ultimate career goals. Pertaining to direct patient care, the MSN prepared NP can do the same things a DNP prepared NP can. Similar to the way an ADN prepared RN can do the same skills as a BSN prepared RN.

Frequently Asked Question: Will the DNP eventually be required? Maybe. There have been a few pushes nationally to require the DNP as entry to NP practice, but at this time, it has not been successfully implemented. The National Organization of Nurse Practitioner Faculty (NONPF), is one of the primary leaders encouraging this to be the case. To learn more, visit their website, https://www.nonpf.org/page/DNP_NPCompetencies.

Goodness of Fit: Program Formats

Once you understand the difference between the master's and doctoral degrees, the next step is choosing the program structure that fits your starting point. Nurses who already hold a Bachelor of Science in Nursing (BSN) typically enter one of two types of programs: a BSN-to-MSN pathway or a BSN-to-DNP pathway.

A BSN-to-MSN program allows you to complete your master's degree in two to three years of full-time study. After graduation, you are eligible to sit for your national certification exam and begin practicing as an NP. Many nurses choose this route because it allows them to start working sooner, gain experience, and decide later whether they want to return for a Doctor of Nursing Practice degree.

A BSN-to-DNP program combines both the master's and doctoral coursework in one continuous plan of study. These programs usually take three to four years full-time and are designed for students who want to complete their terminal degree in one step. While this option requires more time and more financial commitment upfront, it removes the need to stop and reapply later for a separate doctoral program.

Some schools also offer what is known as a "stop-out" option. This allows BSN-to-DNP students to pause their studies once they finish the MSN portion, sit for certification, work as an NP, and then return later to finish the remaining DNP requirements. This structure recognizes that careers and life circumstances sometimes change during graduate study and gives students more flexibility.

There are also a few less common variations. For example, some schools offer ADN-to-DNP tracks for associate degree nurses who want a single, streamlined progression. Others offer entry-level master's programs for students with a non-nursing bachelor's degree, but those graduates still need to pass the NCLEX before pursuing an NP specialty. Most readers will not need these alternatives, but it is important to understand that program design can look different from school to school.

The key decision is deciding whether you want to enter practice sooner through a master's program or commit to the full doctoral pathway now. Both options lead to NP certification and licensure, but the timing, cost, and long-term goals will determine the best fit.

The chart below provides a side-by-side comparison so you can quickly see how the two-degree options differ in length, cost, flexibility, and long-term focus.

Category	Master of Science in Nursing (MSN)	Doctor of Nursing Practice (DNP)
Purpose	Prepares you to become an NP and enter advanced clinical practice	Prepares you for NP practice plus additional training in leadership, systems change, and evidence-based practice
Time to Complete	~2–3 years full-time (longer if part-time)	~3–4 years full-time (may extend to 5–6 years part-time)
Career Entry	Allows you to become licensed and start working as an NP sooner	Includes NP preparation and the terminal degree in one continuous program
Certification and Licensure	Eligible to sit for national NP certification and apply for state NP licensure	Eligible to sit for national NP certification and apply for state NP licensure

Category	Master of Science in Nursing (MSN)	Doctor of Nursing Practice (DNP)
Depth of Training	Focused on advanced clinical care and NP role transition	Includes clinical care plus leadership, policy, quality improvement, and advanced population health
Cost	Lower overall tuition and fewer semesters	Higher total cost due to extended coursework and clinical/scholarly requirements
Flexibility	Can complete MSN now and return later for DNP if desired	One-step option that eliminates the need to reenroll later
Best Fit For	Nurses who want faster entry to practice or need a shorter, more affordable route	Nurses who already know they want a terminal degree, a leadership role, or academic options
Common Misunderstanding	"MSN NPs are less qualified." Not true. MSN and DNP NPs take the same certification exam.	"DNP is required to practice." Not yet. Both degrees are valid for NP licensure.

Experience Before NP School

Most future NPs benefit from at least one to two years of clinical practice before entering graduate school. That time strengthens clinical judgment, improves communication with patients and teams, and makes coursework and clinical rotations more meaningful. Many programs list one to two years of RN experience as "preferred" (AACN, 2023) and some applicants accumulate more before enrolling. There is no single nursing background that guarantees success; every applicant brings strengths and learning gaps. A nurse from labor and delivery may feel comfortable with women's health content but needs more study time in chronic disease management. That balance is normal.

If you plan to pursue women's health, then labor and delivery, or postpartum, experience in these fields is extremely helpful for both learning and clinical placement. The same pattern applies in other specialties: emergency department experience supports preparation for emergency care, and ICU or step-down experience supports acute care practice.

If you are unsure how much experience is recommended, check the programs on your list. Review their admissions language, ask an advisor, and, if possible, speak with current students. Your goal is to begin graduate study with a solid enough foundation that you can focus on advanced learning rather than catching up on core bedside skills.

Faculty Tip

In general, I support the notion that 1-2 years of nursing experience is optimal before starting an NP program. I do not find that there is one type of nursing more beneficial than the other. I have not had good experiences with NP students with less experience than this. Believe me I have tried. They might pass school, but they are generally not strong clinicians afterwards. I find this especially true for those that did RN as a second degree and rapidly completed nursing school, just to get directly to NP school. Just my humble opinion.

If You Plan to Teach

Many nurses seek the NP degrees because they plan to teach later. If that is you, then plan your degree with your future teaching environment in mind. Community and teaching-focused universities often hire master's-prepared faculty for many roles, and they value the DNP for clinical teaching and leadership. Research-intensive universities, however, typically require a PhD for tenure-track positions because their core work centers on original research and grant-funded scholarship (AACN, 2019). If you want to stay primarily clinical and teach in practice-based programs, the DNP is often the best fit. If your goal is academic research and publication, the PhD is the usual path.

A helpful rule of thumb: when possible, hold one degree higher than the level you plan to teach. If teaching is part of your career plan now or later, review degree requirements on faculty job postings and program websites and speak with department chairs. Aligning your education with likely hiring criteria saves time, tuition, and frustration.

Category	Master of Science in Nursing (MSN)	Doctor of Nursing Practice (DNP)	Doctor of Philosophy in Nursing (PhD-Nursing)	Doctor of Education (EdD)
Primary Focus	Advanced clinical practice and preparation for advanced nursing roles	Clinical leadership, evidence translation, and quality gains	Original research and creation of new nursing knowledge	Educational leadership, curriculum design, and pedagogy
Purpose in Academia	Entry-level qualification for teaching in associate and some bachelor's programs	Preparation for clinical teaching, simulation, or practice-based faculty roles	Preparation for tenure-track, research-intensive, or graduate-level teaching positions	Preparation for leadership in education, curriculum innovation, and administration
Typical Teaching Levels	ADN and BSN programs	BSN, MSN, and DNP programs (clinical and applied focus)	BSN, MSN, PhD, and DNP programs (research and theory focus)	BSN and MSN programs, or academic administration

Category	Master of Science in Nursing (MSN)	Doctor of Nursing Practice (DNP)	Doctor of Philosophy in Nursing (PhD-Nursing)	Doctor of Education (EdD)
Type of Scholarship Emphasized	Application of evidence-based practice	Translation of evidence into clinical/educational settings	Generation of new research, theory, and publications	Development of teaching strategies, learning assessment, and faculty leadership
Research Requirement	Capstone or thesis focused on clinical or educational practice	DNP project showing evidence use and results	Dissertation with original research adding new knowledge	Dissertation or applied project in educational theory or leadership
Tenure Eligibility	Rare (mostly teaching-focused institutions)	Possible in practice-oriented or non-research institutions	Common in R1 or R2 research universities	Possible in education-focused universities or schools

Selecting a Quality Program: Accreditation, Format, and Clinical Placement

When choosing a program, start with finances: don't overpay. Select a school that fits both your budget and your learning style. Ask yourself whether you thrive with in-person interaction or prefer flexible online coursework. Verify whether classes are synchronous (set meeting times) or asynchronous (self-paced). Since COVID-19, many institutions have adopted hybrid models that combine both. If you plan to study fully online, confirm that you will still have access to libraries, writing support, faculty office hours, and academic advising.

Equally important is accreditation. Programs accredited by the Commission on Collegiate Nursing Education (CCNE) or the Accreditation Commission for Education in Nursing (ACEN) ensure you will be eligible for national certification after graduation (CCNE, 2024; ACEN, 2024). Without accreditation, you could finish a degree that does not qualify you to sit for boards. Program accreditation is not the same as "state approval" or institutional accreditation. If CCNE or ACEN is not listed on the program website, stop and verify before you apply.

Another critical factor is clinical placement. Some schools secure preceptors and clinical sites for you. Others provide "support" but still expect you to find your own placements. Read the fine print. Look for clear language such as "school-arranged clinical placement" rather than vague terms like "assistance provided." If you are responsible for securing your own preceptor, build in time, networking effort, and potential travel costs. For some students, clinical placement is the single biggest stressor of NP school, not the coursework.

Will you have to pay for a preceptor? Maybe. Some schools will pay the preceptor but may charge you a fee. Or the fee could be included in your student fees. There are also private services that are outside of the school to assist students with finding preceptors. When using those services, you are paying the agency, who then finds and pays a preceptor. This is discussed in more detail in Chapter 4 but estimate approximately $1,500-$3,000 per rotation (NPHub, 2025). Most professional NPs agree that it is our professional duty to mentor NP students. Others, well, they want the money. Just be aware, it does take time to mentor the student. It slows you down. It's hard sometimes.

Faculty Tip

Be aware that online schools have limits about where you can do your clinicals. It is based on your state of residence and the states in which the school has "permission" from the Board of Nursing to allow students. They do not want competition for their clinical sites. If you are military, you need to be careful about this also. Ask specifically in which states you are allowed to do hours.

Applications and Interviews

Most programs use online application systems. Even when requirements vary, competitive applications share the same core elements: a clear, well-written personal statement, a professional resume or CV, strong references, and error-free submission materials. Follow every instruction exactly, including word limits, document format, and file naming. Faculty reviewers notice details. An application with typos, missing items, or ignored directions signals concern about professionalism and readiness for graduate-level work.

What strengthens a graduate nursing application:

- A personal statement that explains your "why" with clarity and focus

- A resume or CV that highlights clinical experience, leadership, and certifications

- References who can speak to your judgment, reliability, and professionalism

- Clean formatting, correct grammar, and documents submitted exactly as requested

- Early submission (i.e., well before the deadline, not on it)

- Professional communication in every email, phone call, and interaction with faculty

A strong personal statement explains why you want to become an NP, why you chose your specialty, and how your experience has prepared you for advanced study. Choose recommenders who can speak directly to your clinical judgment, reliability, and character, not just people with impressive titles. Indicate specific examples and specific times you have observed NPs doing their work. Faculty can spot the people lying.

Some schools include interviews. Even when interviews are not required, it is wise to attend an information session or meet a faculty member. You are evaluating the program as much as they are evaluating you. During interviews, be ready to describe what you have done to understand the NP role beyond internet research, the salary range you expect in your region, how you plan to balance coursework with work and family, and why this program is the right fit. Preparation shows. Use Appendix B: *NP School Interview Preparation Checklist* to review the most common questions and expectations.

Can I Afford It?

Can you afford it? By that I mean, the schools fees and tuition? To work less? To take a similar, maybe lesser salary for a while when you graduate? Let's be very honest here.

Before you enroll, take a hard look at how you will pay for school and how you will live while you are in it. Many students assume loans will take care of everything, but funds can run out if you fail a course, extend your program, or take a leave of absence. If you fail out of NP school, you will still owe the money. If you don't finish NP school, you will still owe the money.

Other considerations: Private v public school? MSN v DNP? What if you can't work? Do you have job potential when you graduate?

Also, effective July 1, 2026, the federal government may limit amounts graduate nursing students can borrow to $20,500 per year and $100,000 total. Private loans cannot be forgiven in public service forgiveness programs either. Be careful here, keep up with the trend.

A simple monthly budget is one of the most effective stress reducers you can put in place. Whether you use an app like Monarch Money or EveryDollar, or prefer pen and paper, the method is less important than consistency. Know your baseline cost of living before you borrow money or accept a job offer later.

To assist, visit Appendix C, *Can I Afford It?* In that exercise, you can spend some time answering these questions and investigating potential scenarios.

Chapter Summary

Choosing the right degree and nursing program requires more than simply deciding to "go back to school." It calls for a clear understanding of what each graduate pathway prepares you for, how long it will take, what it will cost, and how it shapes your future practice. In this chapter, you explored the differences between the MSN and DNP, compared the two main BSN routes into advanced practice, and learned how accreditation, program format, and clinical placement policies can impact your experience from day one.

You also examined how prior RN experience influences readiness for graduate work, and how your long-term goals, including teaching, may affect which degree you choose. The final section shifted from choosing a path to earning your place in it, outlining what makes an application competitive and how to prepare for faculty interviews with confidence.

Your goal is not only to be accepted, but to be intentional about where you train and why. The right program should fit your life, align with your goals, and prepare you to practice safely and confidently. Use Appendix B: *NP School Interview Preparation Checklist* and Appendix C: *Can I Afford It?* to begin organizing your next steps. In the next chapter, you will learn how to prepare for the academic workload, financial planning, and lifestyle adjustments that support success throughout NP school.

Chapter 3:
Succeeding in the NP Classroom

Before you begin graduate-level nursing coursework, it's important to understand that NP school is not only an academic commitment, but a life commitment. The program will demand time, energy, money, focus, and support, and those demands will unfold alongside everything already happening in your world. This chapter is designed to help you enter NP school prepared rather than surprised.

We'll begin by looking at the real-world factors that influence student success, including time management, financial planning, work–life balance, and the reality that life events will continue while you are in school. Once that foundation is set, we'll move into the academic systems that support strong performance, including university policies, technology readiness, and the writing and communication skills expected at the graduate level.

You'll also learn what to expect from the three core graduate courses known as the "3 Ps," how NP exams are structured, how to manage test anxiety, and what it means to complete a scholarly or capstone project before graduation.

By the end of this chapter, you will be able to:

- Identify the life adjustments and support systems needed to succeed in NP school.

- Use orientation and university resources strategically to strengthen academic readiness.

- Demonstrate preparedness in academic writing, technology use, and professional communication.

- Describe the purpose and content of the "3 Ps."

- Apply effective study and test-taking strategies, including techniques for managing test anxiety.

- Explain the role of the scholarly or capstone project in completing your graduate degree.

The goal is to build enough stability and structure that you can fully engage with the learning, clinical reasoning, and professional growth ahead. Many faculty say, "You will get out of it what you put into it." I agree. Your future patients deserve a clinician who has had enough time to learn the material well.

Preparing Your Life for the Demands of NP School

School Happens Inside Real Life

Graduate school does not pause the rest of your world. Birthdays, school plays, shift changes, aging parents, and unexpected illnesses will all happen while you are completing advanced coursework. The goal is not to create a perfect life before you begin, but to enter the program with realistic expectations and a support system that understands what you are taking on.

Interruptions Will Happen

Emergencies, illnesses, and family crises are not a matter of if, but when. When something serious occurs, communicate early and clearly with your faculty. Email first, then follow up by phone always. Always keep written records of what was discussed. Most instructors will work with you within reason, but they cannot help if they do not know what is happening. Never assume a policy is flexible unless you have confirmed it with the person teaching the course. Refer to and utilize the exact instructions in your university policy, program handbook, and course syllabus.

Time Management Is a Clinical Skill

Graduate-level work requires time that does not magically appear. Assignments take longer, readings are denser, and clinical preparation adds a second workload on top of life and employment. Time management is not just an academic skill; it is a patient-safety skill. If you are constantly rushed now, that pattern will follow you into practice. Treat your calendar like a clinical tool. Schedule study blocks, rest, and non-negotiable family time. Protect them as you would a medication pass or a sterile procedure. You could truly hurt someone if you are not fully vested in learning this content.

Balancing Work and School

Many NP students continue working while completing their graduate education, especially in the early semesters. Some thrive with reduced hours, while others discover that full-time work and graduate study are not compatible. Schools rarely ask about your job. Employment is never accepted as a reason for late work or missed deadlines. Let me say that one more time – Your job/work is NEVER an appropriate reason for late work – period. If your life is already stretched thin, it may be wise to delay enrollment rather than to risk burnout, failure, or unsafe clinical performance. You will get out of NP school what you can put in. Your future patients deserve a clinician who has had enough time to learn the material well.

Orientation Readiness

Whether you have already attended orientation or it is still ahead, use Appendix D: *Orientation Readiness Checklist* to confirm that you have the essentials covered before coursework begins. Every program structures its onboarding differently, but most cover the same core information. Reviewing these items now can help prevent confusion, missed deadlines, or last-minute stress once classes are underway.

Orientation is your first opportunity to understand how your program operates. Treat it like the handoff report before a clinical shift; you are receiving the information you will need to perform safely and efficiently. Take notes, ask questions, and clarify anything that seems uncertain. This is the time to learn how communication flows within your program, who your main points of contact are, and how support systems such as advising, tutoring, and counseling are accessed.

Many students underestimate how much orientation shapes their confidence. Those who leave orientation knowing where to find resources and whom to contact when problems arise adjust more smoothly to graduate-level expectations. Approach orientation with curiosity and attention rather than passivity. The effort you invest in understanding your program early on will pay dividends once assignments, exams, and clinical requirements begin.

Review University and Departmental Policies

Once you are accepted into your university and NP program, your priority should be to review both institutional and program-specific policies. These documents explain your rights, responsibilities, and the academic and personal support available to you. Pay close attention to policies on attendance, grievance procedures, learning accommodations, and professional conduct.

Become familiar with the university resources included in your tuition [or what resources are lacking]. Many students overlook services such as writing centers, tech support, tutoring, citation management tools, and full access to academic journals and databases. These supports can make an enormous difference in your academic performance. Know where they are and how to use them. If there are gaps, you may need to factor in more money in your budget.

Your department should provide a catalog or curriculum plan that lists all degree requirements, including course numbers, credit hours, course descriptions, and when courses are typically offered. It should also clarify expectations for scholarly or capstone work, along with the total number of clinical hours required for graduation. The school should also describe the types of clinical settings permitted as it relates to the course/rotation as well as information on how to secure a preceptor. Remember: clinical hour requirements vary by school and specialty.

Technology Readiness

Graduate-level nursing programs expect students to arrive with a basic level of technological competence. The best time to get comfortable with the required tools is before the first assignment is due. Your goal is not to master every system in advance, but to eliminate preventable frustration once the academic workload increases.

Start by reviewing your program's technology requirements in the student handbook or on the university website. Confirm whether a particular operating system, software package, or device is recommended. If your current laptop is slow, outdated, or unreliable, upgrade it now rather than risking a crash during coursework. A functional computer is not an optional convenience in graduate school; it is an essential academic tool.

Most NP programs rely on a learning management system for assignments, a cloud-based file system for document sharing, and standard software for papers and presentations. Many universities offer free student access to the platforms they require, so check before you purchase anything. Confirm whether your program provides free access to academic tools such as Microsoft Office, Grammarly, EndNote, or Zotero before buying individual subscriptions. If your school offers a technology orientation module, complete it early. The hour you spend learning how to upload a file or format a document before classes begin will save you far more time later.

Once your student email account is activated, use it consistently and professionally. Most faculty are required to communicate only through official student email accounts, and messages sent through personal accounts are often ignored for privacy and security reasons. Treat email as part of your professional record. Write clear subject lines that include the course number, use full sentences, and allow one to three business days for a reply. Patient information should never be included in written communication, even when assignments involve clinical topics.

Faculty Tip

Develop a naming system for your papers. I recommend including your last name, the date, the course number, and a brief key word of the assignment. If you just upload or email papers without that it is hard for both you and the faculty to identify later because there are so many. Also, when you send an email to faculty, include your last name and course in the subject line. Again, makes it easier for everyone to stay organized.

Strong technology habits do not make you a better clinician, but they do make you a more efficient graduate student. Reliable tools, organized files, and professional communication will free up time and attention for what matters most: learning to think and practice at the advanced level.

Academic Writing Essentials

Graduate nursing programs expect clear, professional, and well-organized writing. Most students enter NP school comfortable with clinical documentation, but academic writing is a different skill. Expect to write discussion posts, reflection papers, literature reviews, and evidence-based assignments. These require full sentences, correct grammar, logical structure, and accurate citation of sources.

Faculty Tip

Writing with proper grammar is my #1 pet peeve. Yes, as a nurse practitioner you do have to write letters to insurance companies, there is a purpose! People write today as if they are texting. This is GRADUATE SCHOOL! Learn to use a comma properly. Sadly, I even must explain to my GRADUATE students that, "A paragraph is like a hamburger – it has the main burger (meat), and then a bun on top, condiments, and a bun on the bottom." (I got that from my sister who teaches second grade). But it's true. A paragraph has a main idea (the burger), an opening remark (bun on top), supporting information (condiments), and a concluding remark (bun on the bottom). Get it together friends. An if your cover page is not correct APA, I'm already angry when grading your paper. Think about it.

Strong writing is not about sounding scholarly. It is about communicating ideas clearly, supporting your points with evidence, and following the formatting style required by your program. Whether your school uses the Americal Psychological Association [APA] Manual (2020), the American Medical Association [AMA] Manual of Style (2020) or an internal template, learn the expectations early and use them consistently. APA and AMA style guides are periodically updated, so always follow the edition and format your university specifies rather than relying on examples from older books or online templates.

If writing is not your strength, or if English is not your first language, build support now. Most universities offer writing tutors, librarian guidance, workshops, citation guides, and software tools. Use them before you feel overwhelmed, not after.

Minimum writing skills expected in NP school include:

- Organizing a paper with an introduction, body, and conclusion
- Citing sources correctly within the text
- Creating an accurate and complete reference list
- Proofreading for clarity, grammar, and flow before submission
- Writing in a professional tone rather than conversational language

Before courses begin, gather the tools that will support you throughout your program:

- Your school's official writing or citation guide
- A sample paper or template provided by your program
- Access to your university's writing center
- Proofreading software such as Grammarly or Microsoft Editor
- A citation manager such as Zotero, EndNote, Mendeley, or RefWorks

Academic writing improves with practice, feedback, and revision. Developing your writing process now will make future assignments less stressful, especially when several are due at the same time.

Writing Support Team

Academic writing improves with practice, feedback, and revision, and most successful graduate students do not do it alone. Think of your writing support as a team rather than a single resource.

You need two types of editors:

1. A content editor: Someone knowledgeable in nursing or healthcare who can check accuracy, logic, and alignment with clinical evidence.

2. A layperson editor: Someone unfamiliar with the field who can confirm that your paper makes sense to an educated reader. If they can understand your argument, your writing is clear.

Many universities offer free writing-center feedback or light editing. If you plan to hire a professional editor, allow enough time for turnaround. Same-day results are not realistic.

Here are some key considerations before hiring an editor:

- Clarify what level of editing is included, such as proofreading or developmental editing

- Check turnaround times and whether rush fees apply

- Request a sample edit or test paragraph

- Confirm they are familiar with nursing terminology and APA or AMA style

- Ask whether they check citations or only grammar

- Budget realistically. The more technical the paper, the higher the editing cost

Students often ask where to find reliable editors. The following chart highlights major services, what they offer, and what you can expect to pay.

Service	Services Offered	Typical Cost*	Website
Scribbr	Proofreading, structure checks, citation editing	~ $0.017 per word (example: 8,000 words ≈ $161 for 7-day turnaround)	scribbr.com
Oxford Editing	Academic manuscript editing	3.5–20¢ per word (~$8.75–$50 per page)	oxfordediting.com
Wordvice	Academic English editing and proofreading	$0.023–$0.044 per word	wordvice.com
Science Journal Editors	Copy and developmental editing for research manuscripts and theses	~ $0.089 per word (minimum $200)	scienceje.com
Editor World	Academic editing with word-count pricing	~ $0.021 per word	editorworld.com

As you progress, you will also rely on plagiarism checkers, citation software, and AI-assisted writing tools. The next section explains how to use these responsibly, so your work remains both ethical and academically sound.

Academic Integrity: Plagiarism and the Use of AI

Graduate school requires original thinking, accurate citations, and honest academic work. Plagiarism is not limited to copying and pasting. It can also include paraphrasing too closely without credit, reusing work you submitted in a previous course without permission, or turning in writing created by another person or by AI (Artificial Intelligence). Most students who run into plagiarism issues did not intend to cheat. They were rushing, confused about the rules, or unsure how to cite correctly. Asking for help early is always better than repairing a problem later.

Most universities use plagiarism-detection software that scans assignments against published sources and past student work. Faculty review these reports and can usually tell the difference between a formatting error and intentional dishonesty. Similarity scores under about 3–5 percent are generally acceptable, but thresholds vary by school. If your report shows a higher percentage, review the highlighted sections, correct any missing citations, and resubmit when possible. If something feels uncertain, ask before you submit. That one question can save you from a formal academic review.

AI tools such as ChatGPT, GrammarlyGO, and Google Gemini are now part of academic life. They can be used for brainstorming, organizing ideas, improving grammar, or clarifying wording. However, using AI to generate full paragraphs, write assignments, or create citations that you then submit as your own is considered a violation of academic integrity. If you use AI for limited support, some universities require that you disclose this at the end of your paper. A simple note might read: "Author's Note: Portions of this paper were assisted by ChatGPT for grammar and organization review. All final content and analysis reflect the author's original work." These expectations align with national guidance on ethical AI use in nursing education published by the National League for Nursing (2024).

Here are the most common academic integrity expectations in NP programs:

- All submitted work must be your own unless a group assignment is clearly approved.

- All sources, ideas, quotes, and data must be cited using the required format, usually the newest APA edition.

- Reusing your own work for a new assignment without permission counts as self-plagiarism.

- Patient information or clinical identifiers must never appear in coursework.

- Academic misconduct can lead to failed assignments, course failure, probation, or dismissal, depending on the situation.

A simple rule: AI can support your thinking, but it cannot think for you. If you did not analyze it, organize it, or write it yourself, it should not appear in your paper.

Examples of acceptable AI use:

- Brainstorming topics or outlines
- Checking grammar, sentence flow, or clarity
- Creating study questions or practice scenarios

Examples of unacceptable AI use:

- Submitting AI-generated writing as your own
- Using AI to complete discussion posts, papers, or exams
- Letting AI create sources, citations, or data
- Copying AI text into your work without editing or citation

Faculty Tip

AI can help you think and get organized, but it cannot replace your judgment. Faculty look for your voice, your analysis, and your clinical reasoning. It is easy to spot students who simply do not know the content or have no ability for critical thinking. Be sure to check your school and course policies on use of AI.

Reviewing a Curriculum and Syllabus

A curriculum is the official map of your NP program. It shows all required courses, how they fit together, and how they align with program learning objectives and national advanced-practice competencies.

This information should appear in the university catalog. Once you are formally admitted, schools generally do not change your curriculum retroactively. You usually graduate under the catalog year in which you entered. Read the fine print, since some institutions allow limited updates.

A syllabus is the official contract for an individual course. It lists required materials, grading criteria, due dates, and course objectives. Any changes after the term begins must be communicated in writing with proper notice. The syllabus also specifies communication methods, academic appeal processes, and professional expectations. Review it carefully and ask questions on the first day.

The "3 Ps"

In NP education, faculty often refer to three core graduate-level courses as "The 3 Ps": Pathophysiology, Pharmacology, and Physical Assessment. These courses form the academic foundation for advanced practice and are strong predictors of clinical success.

Many NP students use supplemental resources to strengthen their understanding before starting the program or to reinforce weak areas during the semester. Several well-known education companies offer review modules, question banks, or practice exams aligned specifically with the 3 Ps.

Faculty Tip

If you want to get a jump start on content prior to starting your NP program, the 3Ps is a great place to start. There are courses online you can take a ahead of your program. Start reading and get in gear so that you can more easily digest the content that often comes hard and fast. In the next table, there are resources to explore.

Service	Services Offered	Brief Overview
Barkley & Associates	Diagnostic Readiness Tests (DRTs) + Certification Review (live, webinar, home-study)	Offers 100-question "3 Ps" diagnostic exams with rationales to assess readiness. Also provides full NP certification prep across all specialties.
Fitzgerald Health Education Associates	NP certification review courses, on-demand modules, university integration	Includes live, livestream, and on-demand review courses. Their resource library contains pharmacology, diagnostics, and disease-based modules related to the 3 Ps.
APEA (Advanced Practice Education Associates)	Live review courses, question banks, "3 P Exam" prep tools	Known for high pass rates. Their "3 P Exam" assesses advanced pathophysiology, pharmacotherapeutics, and physical assessment knowledge.

For detailed study strategies for each of the 3 Ps, including step-by-step learning methods and faculty guidance, see Appendix E: *Study Tips for Pathophysiology, Pharmacology, and Physical Assessment.*

Test-Taking During Your NP Program

NP exams, whether in coursework or on national certification boards, are designed to assess clinical reasoning rather than simple memorization. Most questions require you to interpret data, apply knowledge to a patient scenario, and select the best response based on standards of care.

You may encounter any of the following formats in program exams, simulation labs, or board exams:

- **Multiple-choice:** Single best answer based on current evidence

- **Select-all-that-apply:** Requires identifying all correct responses

- **Case-based questions:** Full patient scenarios with history, findings, or labs

- **Matching items:** Pairing concepts such as drugs to their side effects

- **Drag-and-drop:** Ordering steps or processes in sequence

- **Hot spot questions:** Clicking on the correct anatomical area or image region

- **Fill-in-the-blank:** Dosage calculations, lab values, formula-based answers

- **Exhibit/Table questions:** Interpreting data from charts, images, or documentation

- **Audio/visual identification:** Recognizing sounds, images, or clinical findings

- **Short-answer responses:** Brief written rationales, SOAP note elements, or care priorities

Multiple-choice questions make up the majority of NP exams. Although they may appear simple, they are designed to test judgment, not guessing or memorized recall.

Each multiple-choice question (MCQ) has three parts:

1. **The stem:** The question or clinical scenario

2. **The correct answer:** The single best response based on current standards

3. **The distractors:** Plausible but incorrect options that test your ability to distinguish "good" from "best"

Example: A patient with congestive heart failure reports leg edema and cough. O_2 saturation is 98% on room air, respirations 22/min. Which lab helps screen and categorize the severity of heart failure?

A. CMP
B. CBC
C. BNP (Correct)
D. LFT

Rationale: BNP (B-type natriuretic peptide) assists in evaluating heart failure severity. The distractor labs are valid tests, but not diagnostic for this condition.

The following strategies will help you approach multiple-choice questions more effectively and with greater confidence:

- Read the stem first and identify what is truly being asked.

- Highlight key words such as first, priority, most appropriate, initial action.

- Trust your first instinct unless you see clear evidence that you misread the stem.

- When two answers seem correct, choose the one that is most correct for safety and scope of practice.

- Think nationally: certification exams follow national guidelines, not regional or local habits.

- Respect team roles: choose answers that reflect the NP scope of practice.

- Use only the information given; do not add assumptions.

- Avoid changing answers unless you clearly misinterpreted the stem.

- Expect visuals, tables, audio clips, and case-based questions; these mirror clinical reality.

Faculty design exams to be valid, reliable, and aligned with objectives. Strong test-takers focus on logic, not luck. Because NP exams are intentionally written to test judgment and clinical safety, the strategies below can help you approach every question more confidently and strategically:

Test Anxiety

Test anxiety is common among NP students and can affect even the most prepared learners. The pressure of high-stakes exams such as pharmacology finals or board certification tests can trigger a stress response that interferes with recall, concentration, and clinical reasoning. Recognizing the signs early and using evidence-based strategies can help you shift from panic to performance.

Test anxiety is an exaggerated fight-or-flight response that activates during exams. Common symptoms include:

- Racing heart, sweating, or shaking
- Nausea or stomach discomfort
- Difficulty focusing or recalling information
- Feeling overwhelmed or suddenly going mentally blank
- Negative self-talk, such as "I am going to fail" or "I am not smart enough"

These reactions do not mean you are unprepared; they simply indicate that the nervous system is overstimulated. With the right tools, anxiety can be managed and reduced. NP students can manage test anxiety more effectively by using the evidence-based strategies below.

1. **Prepare Early and Consistently:** Cramming raises anxiety. Use spaced repetition, short daily study blocks, and timed practice exams to build confidence and reduce uncertainty.

2. **Use Mindfulness and Breathing Techniques:** A few minutes of intentional breathing can reset the nervous system. Try the 4-7-8 technique: inhale for 4 seconds, hold for 7, exhale for 8.

3. **Visualize a Calm and Successful Test Experience:** Mental rehearsal strengthens confidence. Picture yourself focused, calm, and able to recall information clearly.

4. **Challenge Negative Thoughts:** Replace unhelpful thoughts with accurate statements such as:

   - "I have prepared for this material."
   - "I may not know every answer, but I can reason through the question."

5. **Support the Body to Support the Brain:** Take care of your body by maintaining healthy standards for sleep, nutrition, and movement. Some examples include:

   - Aim for 7 to 8 hours of sleep before the exam
   - Eat a protein-based meal and avoid excess caffeine
   - Light exercise or stretching lowers physical tension

6. **Create a Pre-Exam Routine:** Consistent habits signal to your brain that it is time to focus. Examples include listening to calming music, practicing slow breathing, or writing a short encouragement note to yourself.

7. **Know When to Ask for Help:** If anxiety still interferes with performance, seek support early. Most universities offer counseling, coaching, or testing accommodations. Students with diagnosed anxiety disorders can request additional time or quiet testing spaces.

The following tools and programs can help reduce exam-related stress, whether you prefer NP-focused test prep support or general anxiety management resources.

Service	Services Offered	Website
Health Journeys	Guided Imagery for Anxiety	https://healthjourneys.com

Service	Services Offered	Website
NIH Healing Streams Audio Meditations	Audio-guided relaxation for anxiety and panic	https://www.cc.nih.gov/patientlibrary/healing-streams
ANA Well-Being Initiative	Free resilience and mental health resources for nurses and NP students	nursingworld.org

Faculty Tip

Anxiety is real. I have even had to call 911 before because a student was having chest pain during a high-stakes examination. Engage in practice to reduce stress and anxiety. You may consider talking to your own primary care provider about your concerns if they are affecting with your test performance. Don't wait. Start at the beginning of the semester, not when you are desperate to pass.

Capstone and Scholarly Projects

As you progress toward the end of your NP program, you will complete a scholarly or capstone project that demonstrates your ability to apply evidence-based practice to a real problem in healthcare. Whether you are enrolled in an MSN or a DNP program, the purpose of this work is the same: identify a meaningful clinical issue, review and synthesize the evidence, implement a change or intervention, and evaluate the results. Think of it as the bridge between student thinking and advanced-practice clinical reasoning.

Most MSN scholarly projects and DNP practice projects follow a similar developmental path. Students begin by selecting a topic that is relevant, measurable, and feasible within the time and resources available. Once a potential problem is identified, you conduct a literature review to confirm that the issue is truly unmet and that there is justification for change. After faculty approve the proposal, the next steps include implementing your project in a clinical or organizational setting, collecting data, and evaluating outcomes. The process is systematic, rigorous, and designed to strengthen your ability to lead evidence-based change.

If you intend to pursue a doctoral degree, you may be asked early on to consider potential DNP project topics. A strong DNP project addresses a practice-related gap, applies evidence-based interventions, and measures meaningful outcomes. Examples include reducing inappropriate antibiotic prescribing, improving adherence to asthma action plans, increasing screening rates, or enhancing chronic-disease management workflows. Faculty strongly encourage students to choose an advanced-practice issue, not a bedside RN problem. For instance, handoff communication might be appropriate for an RN-focused quality improvement initiative, but it is not a DNP-level practice gap. Likewise, projects built solely around "education" rarely create sustained improvement. Education should be paired with reminders, workflow redesign, policy change, or follow-up mechanisms that address the system as a whole.

The final phase of scholarly and DNP project work—often overlooked early in the process—is dissemination. Sharing your findings is not just a program requirement; it is part of your responsibility as an emerging advanced-practice clinician. Dissemination can take several forms. Some students present a poster at a university research day or state NP conference. Others submit their work to a professional journal or present their outcomes to the leadership team at their clinical site. A well-designed project can lead to policy changes, improved patient outcomes, or even open the door to a job opportunity. Many students are pleasantly surprised by the real-world impact of their project.

Your university will typically provide templates for posters, abstracts, and presentations, especially if you plan to present externally. Organizations such as the American Association of Nurse Practitioners (AANP) and Sigma Theta Tau International offer clear poster guidelines, abstract criteria, and professional presentation tips. University libraries and writing centers may also provide resources on visual design, data display, and scholarly dissemination.

For those considering a doctoral path, additional guidance and practical examples can be found in resources such as The DNP Project Workbook: A Step-by-Step Process for Success (O'Neal & Stevenson, 2021) and The DNP Project Podcast (O'Neal, 2023). These resources offer step-by-step frameworks that help students move from an idea to a completed and disseminated project.

Chapter Summary

Succeeding in NP school requires more than academic talent. It requires planning for the real-world demands that will unfold alongside graduate-level coursework. In this chapter, you explored the practical factors that shape student success, including time management, financial readiness, workload balance, and the importance of communicating early when life interruptions occur. You also learned how orientation, university resources, and proactive communication help you begin the program with confidence.

You examined the academic systems that support graduate-level performance, including technology readiness, writing expectations, and the policies that govern communication, professionalism, and academic integrity. This chapter also introduced the three core graduate courses known as the "3 Ps," outlined how NP exams are structured, and presented test-taking and anxiety-management strategies to support steady academic progress. You also gained an overview of the scholarly or capstone project you will complete near the end of your program and how it prepares you to contribute to evidence-based practice.

If you enter NP school with a realistic schedule, a financial plan, a support system, and an organized approach to academic expectations, you will be able to focus on learning rather than constantly recovering from preventable stress. Without structure, the program will feel harder than it needs to be.

Your goal is not to create a perfect life before school starts, but to build enough stability to fully engage with the learning ahead. Use the readiness tools and checklists in this chapter to evaluate your starting point, then continue to Chapter 4 to learn how clinical rotations work, what to expect from preceptors, and how to prepare for the transition from classroom learning to real-world patient care.

Chapter 4:
How to Excel in Your NP Clinical Rotations

Before you begin your clinical rotations, it's essential to understand what this phase truly involves and how it shapes your transition from student to provider. Clinicals are where classroom theory meets real-world patient care. In this setting, your knowledge, communication, and confidence are tested in real time. This chapter is designed to help you enter that experience with clarity, preparation, and professionalism.

We'll begin by outlining how clinical placements work: who is responsible for finding sites, what to expect from preceptors, and how to stay organized through paperwork, credentialing, and site approval. From there, you'll learn strategies for building and protecting professional relationships, documenting encounters accurately, and demonstrating clinical reasoning through SOAP (Subjective, Objective, Assessment, and Plan) notes and Objective Structured Clinical Examinations (OSCEs).

You'll also gain insight into how competence develops across rotations, using Patricia Benner's (1984) Novice-to-Expert model as a framework for growth. Each section of this chapter provides practical guidance for communication, documentation, and skill development to help you succeed in settings ranging from community clinics to acute care environments.

If you'd like extra preparation tips to make clinicals less stressful, such as organizing your clinical bag or planning meals for long days, see Appendix F: *Clinical Toolkit*. These printable checklists and planning tools are designed to help you stay prepared, organized, and confident throughout your rotations.

By the end of this chapter, you will be able to:

- Explain the structure and purpose of clinical placements in NP education.

- Identify your responsibilities versus your program's in securing and maintaining sites.

- Communicate professionally with faculty and preceptors.

- Document patient encounters accurately using standardized formats.

- Apply strategies for preparing, performing, and reflecting during OSCEs.

- Track your procedural skills and clinical progress effectively.

- Access supporting materials in Appendix F: *Clinical Toolkit* to enhance organization and readiness.

The goal is not simply to survive clinicals, but to enter them as an active learner who is prepared, professional, and ready to grow into the confident, competent nurse practitioner you are becoming.

The Role of Clinicals in NP Education

Clinical placements are the supervised practice experiences where you begin functioning as a provider-in-training, applying everything you learned in the classroom to real patients. A clinical site is the setting where you complete those hours, and a preceptor is the licensed clinician who teaches, evaluates, and signs off on your progress. Together, they form the core of your transition from a student to a safe, independent practitioner.

The purpose of clinicals is simple: to translate theory into competent, real-world care. You will not only perform assessments, practice diagnostic reasoning, and manage treatment plans, but also learn how to think out loud, prioritize multiple problems, communicate with patients, and work within the pace and unpredictability of actual practice.

Before entering clinicals, it helps to understand what they really are, not just what the handbook says they are. At a basic level, clinicals are where you will:

- Apply classroom learning to real patient encounters

- Develop clinical judgment under the supervision of a licensed provider

- Learn the workflow, pace, and culture of different clinical settings

- Build confidence in communicating, documenting, and presenting cases

- Begin forming the professional identity of an NP, not just a student

In a perfect system, every NP program would fully arrange placements, and every student would be matched with an excellent preceptor in their preferred specialty. In reality, placement shortages, competition from other programs, and state-specific rules mean students often need persistence, patience, and networking for a good placement, not just academic strength. Clinicals are both the most rewarding and most stressful part of NP school and understanding the process before you start helps reduce frustration later.

How Placement Works: Roles and Responsibilities

Clinical placement is a shared responsibility between the NP program and the student, but not all schools fulfill their role equally. Accredited programs are expected to secure appropriate clinical sites that align with the student's specialty, meet national competency standards, and provide qualified preceptors. In reality, many schools shift the burden to students, leaving them to cold-call clinics, plead with coworkers, or pay third-party companies for preceptors. Before you enroll, it is essential to understand what a school actually provides versus what it promises in marketing materials.

A well-run program will have a designated clinical coordinator, established affiliation agreements with healthcare organizations, and a documented process for helping students secure sites. They will also verify that each placement matches your population focus. For example, a Family Nurse Practitioner student should be placed in outpatient primary care or community settings, while an Acute Care NP student should not be assigned to pediatrics or long-term care. This alignment is not optional. It is required by accrediting bodies to protect both the student and future patients.

Students also have responsibilities. You are expected to network early, maintain professionalism, follow site policies, complete paperwork on time, and communicate clearly with faculty and preceptors. Being proactive makes it easier to place you, but it should not replace the school's obligation to support you.

A major red flag is any program that tells students, "Clinical placement is your responsibility" or "We cannot guarantee sites." Another warning sign is when current or former students report delayed graduation because they could not find a preceptor. If a program refuses to answer direct questions about placement support, assume the burden will fall on you.

The best programs treat placement like an academic requirement, not a side task. They match you with sites that meet certification standards, oversee preceptor qualifications, and step in if a rotation falls through. The weakest programs leave you on your own and take full tuition anyway. Know the difference before you commit.

A Word on Networking

Networking is not optional in nurse practitioner education. It is one of the most effective ways to secure clinical placements, build professional credibility, and open doors to future employment. The most valuable opportunities in this profession often come not from job boards, but from people who already know your character, work ethic, and clinical interests.

The best time to start networking is the moment you begin NP school. Share your goals with people you already know. Let colleagues, supervisors, and mentors know what specialty you are pursuing and where you hope to practice. When others understand your path, they are more likely to think of you when preceptors, projects, or job openings surface. Many students find their first rotation, mentor, or job because someone simply remembered they were in school.

Professional associations make networking easier. Even as a student, you can join national or state-level organizations to access conferences, scholarships, mentorship, and specialty updates. Common places to start include the American Association of Nurse Practitioners (AANP), the American College of Nurse-Midwives, Sigma Theta Tau International, and your local or regional NP group. Attending a single CE event or chapter meeting can lead to meaningful connections with preceptors, future employers, or peers who are just ahead of you in the program.

Your online presence is part of your network as well. A simple LinkedIn page with a professional headshot, a summary of your background, and your program details signals seriousness and credibility. Many faculty and preceptors look up students before agreeing to work with them, so be sure your digital footprint reflects the provider you are becoming. Update privacy settings on personal accounts, remove anything you would not want an employer to see, and avoid posting patient care content in any format.

Networking is not a transaction. It is the practice of building relationships that last. That means following up when someone gives you advice, sending a thank you note after an interview or introduction, and staying connected with classmates, former preceptors, and alumni. These same people often become future references, collaborators, or supervisors. A strong professional network grows with you and supports every stage of your career, not just your clinical rotations.

Faculty Tip

Your network starts the moment you enter the program. Join your local NP groups (like the state AANP groups) to meet potential preceptors. Have a business card ready with your name, cell, and email. Give that card to everyone you know to help put the word out that you are looking for clinical sites. Start early.

Your Placement Game Plan and Timeline

A successful clinical placement plan does not happen by accident. It requires early preparation, consistent follow up, and an organized system for tracking every email, conversation, and agreement. The earlier you understand the timeline, the fewer delays and last-minute emergencies you will face.

Most NP programs begin clinicals in the second or third semester, but the process of securing sites usually starts long before that. Think of placement as a multi-term project, not a single task. Each semester has its own set of priorities, and staying ahead of them is one of the best ways to protect your progress toward graduation. Most preceptors are booked out at least a year in advanced. For example, I currently have back-to-back students for the next year and a half.

When to Start and What to Do Each Term

During your first term, your only job is to learn how your school handles placements. Know whether sites are assigned, assisted, or entirely student driven. If you are responsible for finding one or more preceptors, begin identifying possible contacts now, even if your rotation is months away. By the end of the first semester, you should already have a list of clinics, providers, or mentors you plan to approach.

During the second term, move from planning to outreach. This is when you begin emailing, calling, or asking colleagues for introductions. Schools often require preceptor information months in advance so they can finalize approval paperwork. Waiting until the term before clinicals is the number one reason students fall behind.

During clinical semesters, your focus shifts to maintaining relationships, confirming schedules, and preparing for the next rotation before the current one ends. Treat every completed placement as part of your professional network. A strong impression now can lead to a job offer later.

Tracking Outreach and Follow-Up

Clinical placement outreach should be documented just like job applications. Keep a simple spreadsheet or tracking document with columns for clinic name, contact person, date of outreach, response status, and follow-up notes. This protects you from duplicated effort and allows you to show your faculty coordinator exactly what steps you have taken if a site falls through. It also helps you avoid losing a lead because an email was forgotten.

If a Placement Falls Through

Rotations can collapse because of staffing changes, illness, or contract delays. As soon as you are notified, email your clinical coordinator and faculty advisor the same day. Include the reason, the effective date, and your placement outreach log. Ask for available alternate sites and the expected reassignment timeline. Continue your own outreach using a short backup list of warm contacts and update the coordinator every three to five business days until reassigned. Keep notes of every call and email so you have a clear record of actions and dates.

Paperwork, Agreements, and Credentialing

Once a site agrees to take you, the administrative work begins. Most schools require a signed affiliation agreement between the university and the clinical site before any hours can be counted. These agreements outline liability, supervision expectations, and legal protections for both parties. They can take weeks or even months to process, especially in large health systems, so submit site details to your school as soon as possible.

In addition to the affiliation agreement, most agencies require credentialing steps such as background checks, immunization records, proof of CPR certification, and HIPAA or OSHA training modules. Some require drug testing or onboarding sessions before you can begin. Start these tasks immediately once assigned. Missing paperwork is one of the most common causes of delayed clinical start dates.

Insurance and Malpractice Coverage

All NP students must carry malpractice insurance during clinicals. Some programs include coverage automatically, while others require students to purchase their own student-level policy. Do not assume your employer's coverage extends to your student role; it does not. Verify coverage details in writing, including start and end dates, coverage limits, and whether telehealth encounters are included.

If you are paying for a personal policy, most student malpractice plans are typically affordable. The peace of mind is worth it. Good coverage protects not only you, but also your preceptor and the clinical site.

How Competence Grows

Like Patricia Benner's classic Novice-to-Expert framework, NP students progress through predictable stages of growth. In the beginning, you function as a novice, relying on structure, checklists, and detailed supervision. As an advanced beginner, you start recognizing common patient patterns and gaining confidence with repeated exposure. The competent stage emerges as you learn to prioritize, plan, and manage complex cases more independently. Over time, proficiency develops, and you begin to integrate experience and intuition into decision-making. Early rotations focus on mastering the fundamentals of history taking and examination, while later ones require diagnostic synthesis, treatment planning, and adaptability. Competence develops through repetition, feedback, and reflection rather than from perfection on the first day.

Paid Preceptorships: When and How to Consider Them

As clinical site shortages increase across the country, paid preceptorship services have become more common. These companies match NP students with preceptors and clinical sites for a fee, often guaranteeing placement within a certain time frame. While they can be a useful safety net, they are not the right fit for every student. Understanding what these services offer, what they cost, and how to evaluate them will help you make an informed decision rather than a rushed one.

What Paid Services Offer and What They Cost

Most paid placement companies maintain a network of clinics and preceptors willing to accept NP students in exchange for compensation. The student pays a fee, and, in return, the company secures the required site, preceptor, and paperwork for a specific rotation. Costs vary widely but often range from 1,500 to 3,000 dollars per rotation. Some agencies charge by the hour, with rates between 10 and 17 dollars per clinical hour NPHub, 2025). Pricing depends on specialty, location, and urgency. Highly competitive rotations such as pediatrics, psychiatry, or women's health often cost more.

Pros and Cons to Consider

Paid preceptorships can prevent delays and allow you to stay on track for graduation. They also reduce the stress of cold calling clinics and competing for limited spots. Students with limited professional networks, those in rural areas, or those attending fully online programs sometimes rely on these services as a last resort.

The main drawback is cost. Students already balancing tuition, books, and reduced work hours may not be able to afford an additional $3,000 per semester. There is also no universal standard for preceptor quality among third-party services. Some students report excellent experiences, while others encounter sites with minimal teaching or high provider turnover.

Confirming School Policy and Site Quality

Before paying any placement company, verify that your school allows third-party preceptors. Some universities prohibit paid arrangements, while others require pre-approval before a contract can be signed. Always check. If your school approves the service, research the site just as thoroughly as if you had found it yourself. Ask about:

- Preceptor qualifications and years of experience
- Number of students taken at one time
- Average patient volume and patient mix
- Whether you can speak with a prior student before committing

You are not only paying for a slot. You are paying for a learning experience that must meet accreditation and board eligibility requirements.

Equity and Access

Paid preceptorships raise real concerns about fairness. Not every student can afford to spend thousands of dollars to access the same clinical education. Some argue that third-party placement creates a two-tiered system: one for students who can pay and one for students who must wait or withdraw.

If cost is a barrier, consider these alternatives before committing to a paid service:

- Ask your school whether hardship funds or tuition grants can be applied to placement fees

- Work with your state NP association, which may maintain free or low-cost preceptor networks

- Request assistance from your faculty or clinical coordinator early, not after a deadline has passed

- Explore whether a nearby school shares placement agreements and can coordinate shared preceptors

- Use alumni connections, former supervisors, or department heads from past jobs as potential leads

Paid placements should be a strategic decision, not a default solution. They are valuable when they prevent program delays, but the best outcome is still a strong, no-cost preceptor relationship built through networking, faculty support, and early planning.

Faculty Tip

Faculty rarely recommend paid preceptors first. However, if they are used, read the fine print of the contracts carefully.

Using Your Workplace as a Clinical Site

Many NP students hope to complete at least one rotation at the organization where they already work. It can be a convenient option, but it is rarely as simple as "I already work here, so they will take me." Even if you are a long-term employee, the institution must credential you as a student, not as staff. That means Human Resources, compliance, and legal departments will process you as an outside learner who requires formal approval, and the timeline can take weeks or even months.

One of my students worked full-time in a large health system and assumed she could complete her women's health rotation in the same department where she was employed. It still took five months for HR and compliance to authorize her as a student. The delay had nothing to do with her job performance, it was simply the standard administrative timeline for onboarding a learner. Plan early and stay persistent.

Before you decide to use your workplace as a clinical site, confirm three things:

1. Whether your program allows students to complete rotations at their place of employment. Some schools permit it, some prohibit it, and others allow it only if the rotation is in a different department.

2. Whether your preceptor must be someone who is not in your reporting line. Many programs require this to avoid role confusion or power imbalance.

3. What paperwork and approvals are required. This may include an affiliation agreement between the university and the organization, proof of student malpractice insurance, HIPAA paperwork, background checks, and/or onboarding modules.

The American Association of Nurse Practitioners (2024) recommends that all clinical sites have a written affiliation agreement with the school. These agreements define supervision, liability coverage, and student expectations. If no agreement exists, your placement cannot move forward, even if a provider has already agreed to take you.

Using your workplace can be a smart clinical strategy, but only if you approach it like any other site. Ask early, follow the required process, and do not assume that your employee status guarantees approval.

Protecting the Preceptor Relationship

Securing a preceptor is only the first step. Once someone agrees to teach you, protecting that relationship becomes just as important as completing the rotation itself. Preceptors volunteer their time, energy, and clinical expertise, often while balancing full patient schedules. The way you show up, prepared and professional, determines whether they view you as a learner they enjoy teaching or an added burden.

Respect their time by arriving early, not just on time. Review the chart before seeing a patient, come with questions ready, and keep your documentation organized. When instructions are given, follow them the first time. If you make a mistake, acknowledge it, correct it, and move forward with maturity.

During patient care discussions, present cases clearly and efficiently. Begin with the chief complaint, summarize key findings, offer your top differentials, and outline your plan. Avoid reading your notes word for word. Focus on concise communication that shows you understand the case and can prioritize next steps.

Small gestures of appreciation matter. A handwritten thank-you note, a sincere expression of what you learned, or a short email at the end of the rotation shows that you understand what they invested in you. Many preceptors keep in touch with former students and later offer mentorship, references, or even job opportunities. Those relationships continue only when respect is mutual.

A strong preceptor relationship is not simply a requirement for graduation. It is the beginning of your professional network. Treat it with care, and you may leave with far more than clinical hours.

Professional Communication with Faculty and Preceptors

Clear, respectful communication is a professional skill as important as any clinical competency. As a nurse practitioner student, you represent yourself, your university, and the profession. The way you communicate, especially when challenges arise, often leaves a stronger impression than any single clinical skill you demonstrate.

If an absence or conflict occurs, notify both your faculty and preceptor immediately and in writing. Do not assume one will inform the other. Use your school email or approved secure messaging platform, confirm receipt, and follow up until the matter is resolved. Keep a brief written record of schedule changes, expectations, and evaluations to prevent misunderstandings and protect your progress.

Before your rotation begins, confirm all contact information for both your faculty and preceptor, including email addresses, phone numbers, and preferred communication methods. Some clinical sites prohibit texting, while others use secure messaging. Clarify expectations during orientation and avoid using personal messaging or social media for professional communication. Never share patient-related information outside approved systems.

Here are a few best practices for maintaining professional communication throughout your clinical rotations:

- **Be proactive, not reactive.** Notify faculty and preceptors of potential conflicts early, well before they escalate.

- **Use professional language.** Emails and messages should be concise, courteous, and free from slang or emojis. Include a greeting, your full name, and a clear purpose for your message.

- **Acknowledge receipt and follow through.** When given instructions, confirm you have received and understood them, and follow up when the task is complete.

- **Respect boundaries.** Avoid contacting preceptors after hours unless it is urgent or they have given permission. Remember that preceptors volunteer their time to teach.

- **Document key communications.** Keep written records of schedule changes, evaluation discussions, or conflict resolutions to ensure clarity and accountability.

- **Handle conflict professionally.** Address misunderstandings privately and respectfully. Seek faculty guidance if needed and avoid airing frustrations publicly or on social media.

- **Express gratitude.** A brief thank-you message after receiving feedback or completing a rotation strengthens professional relationships.

- **Close the loop.** When you complete a request or follow up on a task, notify the person who assigned it. Reliability builds trust.

Documentation You Should Keep

Clinical placement requires more organization than most students anticipate. Your school will maintain official records, but you should always keep your own complete file. If there is ever a delay, a graduation audit problem, or a question about your clinical hours, your personal records become your evidence. Think of this as building a professional paper trail that protects you.

Here are the recommended documents to keep organized and saved throughout your entire program:

1. **Placement Outreach Log:** Keep a record of every site, preceptor, or contact you reach out to. Include dates, names, phone numbers or email addresses, responses, and next steps. This helps you stay organized and proves effort if your program ever needs documentation of your attempts.

2. **Copies of Affiliation Agreements, Clearances, and Approvals:** Save your own copies of everything your school or clinical site requires, including background checks, onboarding modules, liability insurance, immunization records, and official approval letters. Store them digitally and in print so nothing gets lost in transition.

3. **Site Contact List and Backup Options:** Keep a simple list of preceptors, office managers, faculty coordinators, and anyone else connected to your rotation. Add backup sites or contacts so you are never starting from zero if a placement falls through.

4. **Personal Copies of Clinical Hour Verifications:** Download or print your clinical logs at the end of each semester. Systems like Typhon or Exxat can lock after graduation, or you may lose access when your student email expires. Your own copy guarantees proof of hours for certification, licensing, or future employment.

5. **Copies of All Course Syllabi:** Save the syllabus for every course you take, even after the semester ends. Employers, state boards, and certification bodies sometimes request course descriptions years later, especially if you move states or apply for additional licensure. Once you graduate, schools are not always able to retrieve archived syllabi on demand.

6. **Clinical Logs:** Log encounters daily in your program's system (e.g., Typhon or Exxat) and export a PDF at the end of each week. Capture ages, diagnoses, and settings. This helps with accreditation checks and future credentialing. Technology access often ends after graduation, so keep your own archived copies. Use a consistent format for every entry and always protect patient privacy by removing identifiers before saving or sharing logs.

   Note: Many programs provide sample encounter or progress note templates for consistency. If yours does not, there are examples online or request an approved version from your faculty.

7. **SOAP Notes (Your Clinical Reasoning on Paper):** Accurate and organized documentation is one of the most important skills you will develop in clinical training. The standard framework is the SOAP note: Subjective, Objective, Assessment, and Plan, which helps ensure that every patient encounter is clear, concise, and clinically sound.

   - Subjective: What the patient tells you. Include the chief complaint, history of present illness, and relevant past, family, or social history. Use brief patient quotes when appropriate to preserve their voice and context.

- Objective: What you observe or measure. Record physical exam findings, vital signs, and diagnostic results in factual, measurable terms.

- Assessment: Your clinical reasoning. Summarize your working diagnosis and key differentials, including a short rationale that connects the data to your conclusions.

- Plan: What you will do about it. List diagnostic orders, medications with dose and duration, patient education, and follow-up recommendations. Reference current clinical guidelines when outlining care.

SOAP notes are not just paperwork; they reflect how you think. Writing them in real time, avoiding copy-paste habits, and clearly explaining your reasoning show both your understanding of the case and your readiness for independent practice.

Faculty Tip

Clinical systems glitch, emails disappear, and portals close the moment you graduate. Your own saved documents are the only guarantee that you will have the proof you need for certification and future jobs. Be sure to download and save everything before you lose access.

OSCEs: What to Expect and How to Prepare

Objective Structured Clinical Examinations (OSCEs) are performance-based assessments that test your ability to apply knowledge, clinical reasoning, and communication in a standardized environment. Conducting OSCE is expensive for schools and not every NP program uses them. However, you should anticipate some type of high-stakes skill check-off during your program. Their purpose is to prepare you for practice by providing a fair, consistent way to measure competency across all students. OSCEs ensure proficiency in assessment, safety, and communication while building confidence under pressure and strengthening your diagnostic and interpersonal skills. They bridge classroom learning with real-world care, helping you see your progress and readiness for professional practice.

An OSCE typically includes several short stations, each focused on a specific skill or scenario. You will interact with standardized patients portraying consistent conditions while faculty observe and score your performance using structured checklists. Most stations last five to fifteen minutes and may require you to:

- Take a focused history and perform a targeted physical exam
- Explain diagnostic reasoning or present a brief differential diagnosis
- Demonstrate a procedure or provide patient education
- Summarize findings in a SOAP format or verbally communicate a plan

OSCEs are often recorded for later review. Watching yourself afterward helps you identify strengths and areas for growth in communication, organization, and professionalism.

To prepare effectively for your OSCE, focus on six key areas: reviewing essential clinical skills, practicing timing, refining communication, mastering documentation, seeking feedback, and managing stress.

1. **Review key clinical skills and guidelines.** Focus on common complaints such as abdominal pain, chest pain, shortness of breath, and headache, using current evidence-based protocols.

2. **Practice timing and focus.** Rehearse concise histories, targeted exams, and thirty-second case summaries with peers or through mock cases.

3. **Refine communication and empathy.** Use open-ended questions, maintain eye contact, and demonstrate respect and compassion. Faculty assess how you connect with patients as much as what you know.

4. **Review documentation formats.** Be ready to summarize your findings in SOAP format or present them verbally. Organized documentation demonstrates good clinical reasoning.

5. **Seek feedback early.** Participate in practice sessions or simulations that your program offers and apply feedback before the real exam.

6. **Manage stress effectively.** Treat the OSCE as a learning experience. Confidence comes from preparation, not perfection.

Post-exam debriefing is an essential part of learning. Faculty often review recordings or checklists with you to highlight strengths and identify growth areas. Use this feedback to improve your focused physical exams, diagnostic reasoning, and communication. Keep notes in your clinical notebook to track your progress over time.

Procedures and Skills: Build Reps Intentionally

Every clinical rotation offers opportunities to strengthen your procedural skills, the hands-on techniques that define safe and effective patient care. Each site has its own skill expectations that align with program objectives and national standards, ensuring that by graduation, you are proficient in the essential procedures for your specialty.

Progress looks different for every student. Some rotations emphasize suturing or wound care, while others focus on chronic disease management or patient education. Mastery takes time, repetition, and feedback. Simulation labs and Objective Structured Clinical Examinations (OSCEs) provide safe spaces to practice and build confidence before performing procedures independently.

To develop procedural competence, focus on five key strategies:

1. **Use Simulations to Build Confidence.** Practice procedures repeatedly until each step becomes familiar. Pay attention to sterile technique, patient communication, and efficient time management.

2. **Seek Out Local or Continuing Education Opportunities.** Hospitals, simulation centers, and NP programs often host workshops that allow supervised practice before you perform procedures in clinical settings.

3. **Network with Peers and Mentors.** Share opportunities, observe in different specialties, and learn from classmates and colleagues. Collaboration broadens both your experience and professional relationships.

4. **Attend Professional Conferences.** The American Association of Nurse Practitioners (AANP) and other organizations often offer hands-on workshops that strengthen skill proficiency and confidence.

5. **Integrate Evidence-Based Practice.** Pair each new skill with current clinical guidelines. Review USPSTF or AANP recommendations when learning or performing procedures such as Pap smears, joint injections, or wound care (e.g., USPSTF, 2023; AANP, 2024).

Most programs provide a skills checklist to document progress. Treat it as a working record. Note each procedure you observe, assist with, or perform, and include reflections on what went well and what can be improved. Keep a short skills log to track growth over time.

Competence in clinical procedures grows through deliberate practice, constructive feedback, and thoughtful reflection. Each attempt brings you closer to the confidence and consistency expected of an independent nurse practitioner.

Chapter Summary

Clinical rotations are the bridge between classroom learning and real-world NP practice, and success in this phase requires preparation, professionalism, and consistent communication. In this chapter, you explored how clinical experiences are structured, what they are designed to achieve, and how schools, preceptors, and students share responsibility for ensuring safe, meaningful learning. You also reviewed how placements are arranged, why early networking matters, and how to set clear expectations with clinical sites before your first day.

You examined the practical skills that support strong clinical performance, including accurate documentation, effective patient presentations, and the use of standardized frameworks such as SOAP notes and OSCEs. The chapter also introduced strategies for tracking your hours, competencies, and procedural skills, helping you stay organized throughout the semester. Patricia Benner's Novice to Expert model provided a developmental lens for understanding how competence unfolds gradually through repetition, reflection, and steady exposure to increasing levels of complexity.

The chapter emphasized that relationships matter as much as knowledge. Professional communication, gratitude, and reliability strengthen your connection with preceptors and faculty, often opening doors for mentorship, references, and future employment. You learned that clinical success is less about perfection and more about preparation, curiosity, and the ability to adapt under real-world conditions. Students who approach clinicals with humility and initiative gain not only experience but confidence in their emerging clinical judgment.

Use the tools and guidance provided in this chapter to prepare for productive clinical rotations, then continue to Chapter 5 to explore how professional behaviors, emerging leadership skills, and ongoing development deepen your readiness for independent practice.

Chapter 5:
Making the Most of the Final Semester of Your Nurse Practitioner Program

Before you step into professional practice, the final semester of NP school is your bridge between student and clinician. It is the period when academic learning, clinical experience, and career preparation converge. This chapter is designed to help you complete your program with clarity, confidence, and a plan for what comes next.

We'll begin by focusing on certification preparation—how to assess your readiness, organize a study plan, and choose the most effective review tools. From there, we'll shift to building your professional identity through a polished curriculum vitae (CV) and strategic job-seeking techniques.

The chapter also addresses the personal side of transition: balancing family, finances, and lifestyle as you move from graduate student to working NP. You'll explore how to evaluate job location, set healthy expectations, and communicate with loved ones about the changes ahead. Finally, you'll learn how to maintain a professional online presence that supports your credibility and career growth.

By the end of this chapter, you will be able to:

- Develop a structured plan for national certification preparation.
- Create and maintain a professional NP curriculum vitae.
- Apply effective job-seeking and networking strategies.
- Plan for family, lifestyle, and financial transitions after graduation.
- Align your digital and professional identity for career success.

The goal is not simply to finish the program but to transition into practice as a confident, well-prepared clinician who understands both the professional and personal dimensions of beginning an NP career.

Preparing for the Certification Exam

Your preparation for national certification begins the moment you start NP school. Now that you are in your final semester, you have completed the 3 Ps (Pathophysiology, Pharmacology, and Physical Assessment), most of your coursework, and nearly all your clinical hours. You are six months or less away from graduation, which makes this the ideal time to finalize your readiness plan.

Self-Assessment

Take inventory of what you have learned throughout your NP program. Several organizations offer diagnostic tests that mirror the national certification exams. Use these tools to identify weaker areas and create a focused study plan. Spend extra time reviewing the foundational 3 Ps, since those subjects appear frequently on the board exams. Revisit your earlier notes to refresh your knowledge.

To gauge readiness under real exam conditions, consider taking an official practice exam. This may be offered via your school and included in your program, or you could do this activity independently. It will help you prepare, identify weak areas, and then make a formal study plan.

Write a structured study plan with clear goals and review dates, combining full-length practice exams with short daily question sets. Focus intentionally on the areas where you feel least confident instead of spending most of your time on familiar material. Consistency and targeted review build confidence more effectively than last-minute cramming.

Understanding the Candidate Handbook

Once you have a clear sense of your strengths and learning needs, review the official exam handbooks from your certifying organization. Each handbook outlines the test structure, content areas, policies, and credentialing requirements. Reading these early reduces anxiety and helps you plan your preparation timeline.

If you anticipate needing testing accommodations or plan to take your exam internationally, review those procedures as soon as possible, since requests often require documentation and several weeks of processing.

Exploring Test Dates and Registration Timing

Some certifying bodies allow you to begin the registration process before your degree is officially conferred, provided your program verifies completion of all required coursework and clinical hours. Even if you are not yet eligible to test, review available test dates and locations early in your final semester. Most testing vendors release schedules several months in advance, making it easier to estimate when and where you'll sit for your exam. Planning your preferred testing window now allows you to align your study plan with realistic dates and ensures a smoother transition from graduation to certification.

Choosing Your Certifying Body

The table below lists the major nurse practitioner certification bodies by specialty. Identify your population focus and visit the corresponding website to access your official exam handbook, eligibility criteria, and application information.

NP Specialty	Certifying Organization	Certification Offered	Website
Family Nurse Practitioner (FNP)	American Association of Nurse Practitioners (AANP)	FNP-C	www.aanpcert.org
	American Nurses Credentialing Center (ANCC)	FNP-BC	www.nursingworld.org/ancc
Adult-Gerontology Primary Care NP (AGPCNP)	American Association of Nurse Practitioners (AANP)	AGPCNP-C	www.aanpcert.org

NP Specialty	Certifying Organization	Certification Offered	Website
Adult-Gerontology Acute Care NP (AGACNP)	American Nurses Credentialing Center (ANCC)	AGPCNP-BC	www.nursingworld.org/ancc
	American Nurses Credentialing Center (ANCC)	AGACNP-BC	www.nursingworld.org/ancc
	American Association of Critical-Care Nurses (AACN)	ACNPC-AG	www.aacn.org
Pediatric Primary Care NP (PNP-PC)	Pediatric Nursing Certification Board (PNCB)	CPNP-PC	www.pncb.org
Pediatric Acute Care NP (PNP-AC)	Pediatric Nursing Certification Board (PNCB)	CPNP-AC	www.pncb.org
Women's Health NP (WHNP)	National Certification Corporation (NCC)	WHNP-BC	www.nccwebsite.org
Neonatal NP (NNP)	National Certification Corporation (NCC)	NNP-BC	www.nccwebsite.org
Psychiatric-Mental Health NP (PMHNP)	American Nurses Credentialing Center (ANCC)	PMHNP-BC	www.nursingworld.org/ancc
Emergency NP (ENP)	American Academy of Nurse Practitioners Certification Board (AANPCB)	ENP-C	www.aanpcert.org

Comparing AANP and ANCC Exams (FNP & AGPCNP)

For Family Nurse Practitioner (FNP) and Adult-Gerontology Primary Care Nurse Practitioner (AGPCNP) students, two national organizations offer certification. It is worth understanding how they differ.

Feature	AANP Certification	ANCC Certification
Focus	Primarily clinical questions	Combination of clinical, research, and policy questions
Question Format	Four-option multiple choice	Multiple formats (select-all, images, drag-and-drop)
Content Emphasis	Clinical management and pharmacology	Broader scope including theory, research, and leadership
Score Reporting	Pass/fail with a scaled score	Pass/fail with a scaled score
Credential Earned	FNP-C or AGPCNP-C	FNP-BC or AGPCNP-BC

Each exam differs slightly in question style and content balance, so review your specific exam handbook thoroughly before scheduling your test. Both the American Nurses Credentialing Center (ANCC) and the American Academy of Nurse Practitioners Certification Board (AANPCB) are nationally recognized and accredited. While some students describe the ANCC exam as more academic, both are rigorous, evidence-based, and designed to assess safe, competent practice.

If you plan to teach or pursue roles in academia, the ANCC credential may offer advantages because its renewal process recognizes scholarly work and research. The AANPCB renewal, by contrast, emphasizes ongoing clinical practice hours. Most employers do not have a preference between the two, although hospitals with Magnet® status (an ANCC designation) sometimes encourage ANCC certification since it supports their credentialing metrics. Both organizations require continuing education and practice hours for renewal, so reviewing those requirements early helps you plan for long-term professional maintenance.

Looking Ahead to Certification and Practice

You are now entering the final stretch of your NP program. The decisions and preparation you complete during this semester, including reviewing your certifying body's requirements, exploring test dates, and assessing your readiness, set the stage for a smooth transition after graduation. By laying the groundwork now, you will enter the post-graduation phase organized, confident, and ready to begin your career as a certified nurse practitioner.

Once you have your certification goals in motion, the next step is preparing your professional materials for employment. Your curriculum vitae (CV) is the foundation of that process.

Faculty Tip

Students start to get into a panic in the final semester about all the things they need to do. It can be worse if your classmates are even slightly ahead of you in this process. Just know that it is typical for NP graduates to take 6 months to 1 year before everything is in place to start your new role. Just breathe.

Preparing a Curriculum Vitae (CV)

As you transition from student to professional, you will need a curriculum vitae (CV) rather than a traditional resume. Nurse practitioners serve as clinicians, scholars, and leaders, and your CV should reflect that breadth of professional identity. Unlike a resume, which highlights selective experience for a single job, a CV presents a comprehensive record of your academic, clinical, and professional development. To understand how the two differ, consider the following comparison between a resume and a CV:

Feature	Resume	Curriculum Vitae (CV)
Purpose	Summarizes relevant experience for a specific job	Provides a full record of academic, professional, and clinical experience
Length	Typically, 1–2 pages	No formal limit; may extend several pages
Focus	Tailored to one position or specialty	Highlights the full scope of your career and achievements
Content	Job titles, key skills, and brief descriptions	Education, clinical rotations, certifications, publications, presentations, and leadership roles
Audience	Employers seeking specific skill sets	Employers, credentialing bodies, and academic institutions
Tone	Concise and results-focused	Detailed, professional, and scholarly
Update Frequency	Updated during job searches	Updated continuously throughout your career

What Makes a Strong CV

A strong CV is organized, complete, and clear. It communicates your readiness to function as an advanced practice nurse and your ongoing commitment to professional growth. Include the following sections:

- **Education and Certifications:** List degrees in reverse chronological order, including credentials (e.g., RN, MSN, FNP-S, DNP) and certifications such as BLS, ACLS, or specialty credentials.

- **Clinical Rotations and Patient Populations:** Describe the settings, patient demographics, and approximate clinical hours to help employers understand the scope of your experience.

- **Employment History:** Emphasize roles that reflect leadership, sound clinical judgment, and effective teamwork.

- **Scholarly Projects, Presentations, and Publications:** Include examples of evidence-based projects, posters, conference presentations, or journal articles that showcase your professional contributions.

- **Professional Memberships and Volunteer Work:** Include affiliations such as AANP, Sigma Theta Tau, or your state NP association, along with service or advocacy work.

- **References:** Include professional references only if requested. Otherwise, note "Available upon request" and ensure your references have a current copy of your CV.

Keep the design simple and consistent. Use uniform headings, spacing, and fonts. Avoid decorative templates or excessive color; clarity and professionalism should always guide your layout. Your goal is to make it easy for employers, reviewers, or credentialing committees to locate key details at a glance.

Keep a digital version of your CV in both editable (Word) and PDF formats. Store copies in a secure cloud folder, such as Google Drive or OneDrive, so you can update or share them quickly when opportunities arise.

Although your CV should provide a complete record, you can adjust emphasis depending on the opportunity. For example, highlight research and teaching experience for academic applications, or focus on clinical outcomes and certifications when applying for practice positions.

Why a Strong CV Matters for Nurse Practitioners

A CV is more than an application document; it is a professional record that grows with you throughout your career. It reflects your commitment to learning, accountability, and clinical excellence. Nurse practitioners use their CVs for a variety of purposes, including:

- Credentialing and privileging at healthcare organizations
- State licensure and insurance paneling applications
- Academic or clinical teaching roles
- Grants, fellowships, or leadership opportunities

Keeping your CV current allows you to document your professional evolution and highlight your expanding areas of expertise. Once your CV is polished and up to date, begin using it to apply for positions, submit credentialing paperwork, and build your professional network during your final semester.

Should I Do an NP Residency Program?

Residency programs are optional but expanding. Many graduates report higher confidence after structured programs, especially for high-acuity or underserved settings. Balance potential benefits against stipend-level pay, duration, and program quality.

What the Major NP Organizations Say

The American Association of Nurse Practitioners (AANP) maintains that NPs are fully trained at graduation and that residency or fellowship programs should not be required for licensure (Giffith, 2020). In other words, completing your degree program qualifies you for safe, independent practice. However, the option of a residency can provide additional structure and mentorship during the transition from student to clinician.

Reasons to Consider a Residency

A postgraduate program can offer clear advantages for new NPs seeking added support during the transition to practice. Research shows that graduates who complete structured residency or fellowship training often report greater clinical preparedness and confidence (Parkhill, 2010). These programs can be especially valuable for those entering complex or high-acuity settings, such as specialty care, critical care, or underserved community clinics, where mentorship and guided exposure can ease the adjustment period. Some programs even guarantee employment upon completion, offering a direct pathway into a permanent position within the same organization.

Considerations and Limitations

Despite the potential benefits, residency programs come with practical trade-offs. Many offer stipends or reduced pay compared with full NP positions, even though the time commitment can be substantial, often lasting 12 months or longer. Participants may also face limitations on employment options afterward, depending on contract terms or geographic restrictions. Another consideration is program quality. Although the number of residencies continues to grow, accreditation and outcome data remain inconsistent. One study found that nearly three-quarters of surveyed programs were not yet accredited (Kesten, 2020), underscoring the need to evaluate programs carefully before committing.

Connecting Residency to Professional Identity

As you move from student to practicing NP, your professional identity rests on competence, autonomy, and accountability. A residency program can reinforce that identity by bridging the gap between education and independent practice. However, your capability as a clinician does not depend on completing one. A strong NP program should already equip you with the knowledge and skills to begin practice safely and confidently. The choice to pursue residency should therefore depend on your personal learning goals, your practice environment, and your readiness, not external pressure or comparison.

If you're uncertain whether residency training fits your situation, compare your current confidence, goals, and financial readiness using the table below.

If you…	Then a residency might be beneficial
Feel underprepared or have limited clinical exposure	Yes: look for a well-supported program
Plan to work in a high-acuity or underserved setting	Yes: structured support helps with transition
Have multiple job offers and feel confident in your readiness	Maybe skip: begin practice and contract negotiation now

| Have significant financial obligations and cannot delay full earning | Skip: weigh early practice income over residency stipend |

Whether or not you pursue a residency, your next priority is maintaining momentum through licensure, credentialing, and employment preparation.

Faculty Tip

A residency can build confidence, but it is not the only path to feeling ready. Many graduates grow quickly once they begin practicing, especially when they choose supportive teams and ask for help early.

Lifestyle, Support System, and Financial Readiness

The months before graduation are the ideal time to pause and take stock of your life beyond coursework and clinicals. Where you choose to live, apply for licensure, and begin practice will depend not only on your professional goals but also on your personal realities, such as your support system, finances, and lifestyle needs. The answers you uncover now will guide nearly every logistical decision that follows, including where to seek licensure, which jobs to pursue, and how to prepare financially and emotionally for the transition into practice. Planning early allows you to make these moves with confidence instead of reacting under pressure.

Thinking through these factors before you start applying for jobs or submitting license paperwork makes every later step smoother and more intentional. Once you begin the licensure process, switching states or adjusting plans can delay your start date or create unnecessary expense. Taking the time now to clarify your priorities, such as where you want to live, what kind of schedule you can sustain, and what financial stability looks like for you, will help you enter the job market strategically rather than reactively.

Look Ahead Before You Apply

Licensure, credentialing, and job opportunities are often specific to each state. If you anticipate moving, living near family, or seeking a particular lifestyle or cost of living, those choices will influence where and when you apply for licensure. Once the process begins, switching states can delay your start date or add unnecessary expense.

Ask yourself:

- Where do I realistically want to live and practice in the next few years?
- How close do I want to be to my current support system?
- Does my preferred region offer the kind of work setting or schedule I want?

Set Realistic Lifestyle Expectations

Different practice settings have different rhythms. Primary care or behavioral health may offer consistent hours, while urgent care or hospital-based roles often include evenings, weekends, or rotating shifts. Consider how these schedules align with your priorities, such as personal time, study, relationships, health, and other commitments, and decide what level of balance you can maintain.

Even if you live alone, it helps to identify people who can support you during busy or stressful periods. This might include friends, mentors, neighbors, or extended family.

Prompts to explore:

- What does a sustainable weekly routine look like for me?
- How much schedule flexibility do I need for rest, hobbies, or family time?
- Who can I rely on for practical or emotional support during the transition?

Build Financial Readiness

It is common for new graduates to experience a gap of two to three months between completing school and receiving their first nurse practitioner paycheck. Planning ahead can prevent this from becoming a financial strain.

Before graduation:

- Estimate the total cost of certification exams, state licensure, background checks, and malpractice coverage.

- Set aside a transition fund to cover two to three months of essential expenses.

- Review student loan repayment timelines and explore programs for repayment.

- If relocation is likely, include moving and housing expenses in your budget.

Thinking through finances early also helps you compare job offers more accurately. Total compensation, including health insurance, retirement contributions, CME support, and paid time off, often matters more than salary alone.

Plan With Your Support System

Whether your support network includes a partner, family, friends, or roommates, discuss what this next stage will mean for everyone involved. Your new professional responsibilities may shift routines and availability. Being open about your goals helps others understand your needs and support you effectively.

Conversation starters:

- How might my schedule change once I begin working?

- What backup plans do I have for transportation, errands, or family responsibilities?

- What boundaries will I set to protect time for rest and continued learning?

Location Choices

Once you have reflected on your personal needs, support system, and financial readiness, the next step is to decide where you want to build your career. Choosing where to practice is one of the most important decisions you will make as a nurse practitioner. Geography influences nearly every aspect of your professional and personal life, including work-life balance, salary potential, patient population, and scope of practice.

As you evaluate opportunities, consider how commute time, relocation, and community setting may affect your quality of life. A position that looks ideal on paper may become less sustainable if distance, travel costs, or family commitments make it difficult to maintain balance.

Geography also shapes career growth. Your first position often determines your early professional network and future opportunities. Evaluate whether the region supports your long-term goals and desired practice environment.

Review any non-compete requirements early, because distance and duration can limit your options. See "Key Elements of an NP Contract" in Chapter 7 for what to look for and how to negotiate.

Faculty Tip

Most new NPs underestimate how much their support system influences their first year of practice. The students who plan their personal lives as intentionally as their careers adjust faster and stay grounded.

Social Media Presence

In today's digital world, your online image is an extension of your professional identity. Everything you post, from photos to comments, communicates something about who you are as a clinician. Employers increasingly review social media profiles as part of their hiring process, and your digital presence often speaks before you do. As you transition from student to nurse practitioner, it is essential to ensure that your online persona reflects the same professionalism, empathy, and integrity you bring to patient care.

Aligning Your Digital Footprint with Your Professional Identity

Earlier in this book, we discussed the concept of professional identity formation, the gradual process of evolving from "student nurse" to "nurse practitioner." That same transformation should extend to your online presence. The tone, content, and visual presentation of your digital footprint should align with your new professional role. Before posting or sharing, pause to ask yourself whether you would be comfortable with a patient, preceptor, or potential employer seeing it. Consider whether your posts demonstrate the compassion, accountability, and evidence-based mindset expected in advanced practice nursing. Your goal is to cultivate a digital brand that communicates confidence, respect, and trustworthiness.

Conducting a Professional Audit

Before you begin applying for positions or networking professionally, take time to audit your social media accounts. Search your name online to see what appears on the first few pages of results. Review all platforms, including Facebook, Instagram, LinkedIn, and others, and remove or archive posts, photos, or comments that could be interpreted as unprofessional, polarizing, or overly personal. Adjust privacy settings as needed, but remember that privacy controls can change, and screenshots last indefinitely. Update your profile photos to reflect your new professional identity and verify that your credentials are listed accurately. This process ensures that your public image aligns with the clinical credibility and integrity you have worked so hard to build.

Building a Positive Professional Brand

When used thoughtfully, social media can be a valuable tool for career growth. A strong digital presence can highlight your expertise, attract job opportunities, and connect you to a network of like-minded professionals. LinkedIn is often the best starting point. Create or update your profile with a professional photo, a concise summary of your clinical focus, and highlights from your education and experience. Consider joining professional nursing forums, national and state NP associations, or online communities where clinicians share insights, job leads, and continuing education opportunities. Posting or engaging with evidence-based articles, patient education initiatives, or community health events can demonstrate leadership and a commitment to lifelong learning.

Avoiding Professional Pitfalls

Even experienced clinicians sometimes post content that raises ethical or confidentiality concerns. Protecting patient privacy should remain your highest priority. Never share identifying details or clinical scenarios online, even when names or locations are omitted. Avoid venting about workplace frustrations on public platforms and think carefully before engaging in debates that could be seen as unprofessional or politically divisive. Humor, sarcasm, and commentary can easily be misunderstood outside their intended context. The safest approach is to maintain the same tone of respect, discretion, and professionalism online that you would uphold in a clinical environment.

Your Digital Reflection of a Professional Future

Your social media presence is part of your professional portfolio, just like your CV, certification, or reference list. Employers, credentialing bodies, and even patients may look to your online footprint as a reflection of your credibility and maturity. Taking the time now to curate a professional and consistent presence demonstrates readiness for advanced practice and shows that you take your public reputation seriously. The goal is simple: ensure that anyone searching your name, whether a recruiter, colleague, or patient, finds content that reinforces the integrity, confidence, and excellence of your new professional identity.

Faculty Tip

One unprofessional post can outweigh months of strong clinical performance. Protect your reputation now. You worked too hard to let your online presence speak for you in the wrong way.

Avoiding Comparison

Comparison can quietly weaken your confidence during the final semester of NP school. Some classmates will receive job offers before graduation, others may take months to find the right opportunity, and a few may begin residencies or move directly into their dream positions. It can be tempting to ask yourself, "Am I behind?"

Every journey from student to nurse practitioner is unique. Factors such as family responsibilities, clinical experience, financial needs, and job availability all influence the transition. Focusing on your own progress helps maintain perspective and confidence.

Stay Grounded in Your Professional Identity

Your professional identity forms gradually through self-awareness, integrity, and competence. Focus on being prepared for practice rather than on how quickly others secure positions. Even when progress feels slow, each experience strengthens your skills and confidence for the transition ahead.

Recognize That Circumstances Differ

Each graduate's path is shaped by location, specialty, and personal commitments. Urban areas may offer more opportunities but greater competition. Certain NP tracks, such as psychiatric or women's health, often require longer credentialing or hiring processes. Family responsibilities, relocation, or financial realities may also affect how soon you begin your first position. Understanding these differences helps you stay patient with your own progress and supportive of others on theirs.

Cultivate a Supportive Network

Connection helps replace comparison with encouragement. Build relationships with classmates, mentors, and peers who value collaboration and growth. Participate in professional organizations or local NP groups to share insight and normalize the ups and downs of the transition to practice. Surrounding yourself with others who share your goals helps you maintain confidence and motivation.

Turn Comparison into Reflection

When you catch yourself comparing, pause and reframe the thought. Consider what you can learn from another person's path, what personal strengths make your own journey distinct, and what small, intentional steps you can take toward your goals today. Turning comparison into reflection fosters self-awareness and keeps your focus on growth rather than competition.

Celebrate Your Own Timeline

Completing NP school is an achievement that reflects dedication and resilience. Whether your first position begins next month or next year, you have already succeeded. Take time to rest, reflect, and appreciate how far you have come. Your path into practice will unfold at the pace that fits you best.

Graduation Celebrations

You have worked hard, so take time to celebrate it. Completing NP school is no small achievement. Every clinical hour, paper, and late-night study session has led you here. Pause to savor this moment and honor the transformation from student to nurse practitioner.

Graduation is more than a ceremony; it is a celebration of perseverance, purpose, and growth. Whether you are walking across the stage or celebrating from home, share this joy with those who supported you, including your family, classmates, mentors, and the patients who inspired your journey.

One favorite tradition among graduates is taking photos together. A simple cap-and-gown selfie, a white coat picture, or a group shot with classmates captures the spirit of the occasion. These images become a reminder of the hard work, laughter, and friendships that shaped this chapter of your professional life.

As you celebrate, take a quiet moment to reflect. You did not just complete NP school; you grew into the clinician you were meant to be. Allow yourself to feel gratitude, pride, and peace as you step forward into practice.

Chapter Summary

Completing the final semester of NP school involves much more than finishing your last clinical hours. It requires a focused plan for certification, early employment preparation, and your overall transition into professional practice. In this chapter, you explored how to assess your readiness for the national certification exam, organize an efficient study schedule, and select trusted review tools to strengthen your confidence before test day.

You also prepared for your next professional steps by developing a comprehensive curriculum vitae and applying strategic networking and job search techniques. The chapter then guided you through the personal dimensions of this season, including planning for family, finances, and lifestyle changes, evaluating potential job locations, and maintaining a professional online presence.

Together, these steps position you to enter practice with clarity, competence, and confidence. Your goal is not only to graduate, but to transition successfully into the nurse practitioner role you have worked toward.

Chapter 6:
Interviews, Credentialing, Contracts & More

The months prior to and after graduation involve a series of critical steps—certification, licensure, credentialing, and regulatory approvals—that determine when and how you can actually begin practicing. This chapter is designed to help you move through that transition with clarity, organization, and realistic expectations.

Before that happens though you will need to finalize your national certification plan: understanding what your exam requires, using the candidate handbook as your primary guide, selecting review courses and tools, and building a focused, blueprint-aligned study schedule. From there, the chapter walks you through applying for jobs, interviews, and contracts. Then, we will discuss the details of state NP licensure, maintaining your RN license, and planning for the varying timelines and requirements that each Board of Nursing may impose.

You will also learn how credentialing works at the employer and payer level, including what hospitals, clinics, and insurance companies verify before granting you privileges and the ability to bill for services. Practical guidance on obtaining your National Provider Identifier (NPI) and DEA registration is included so you can prescribe and document within legal and regulatory standards. The chapter concludes by explaining how state practice laws and collaborative agreements shape your day-to-day scope of practice and professional autonomy.

By the end of this chapter, you will be able to:

- Finalize a realistic, blueprint-aligned plan for national NP certification.

- Explore job opportunities and determine what should be in your NP contracts.

- Navigate state NP licensure requirements, forms, and expected processing times.

- Explain the purpose and process of organizational credentialing, NPI assignment, and DEA registration.

- Recognize how state practice laws and collaborative or supervisory agreements shape your scope of practice as a new nurse practitioner.

The goal is to enter practice fully authorized, well-prepared, and confident in your next steps. When you have a study plan, a job secured, and understand the certification, licensure, credentialing, and regulatory processes before you begin, you can move through this transition with far less stress and far greater clarity. Each step brings you closer to practicing independently, safely, and with the professional grounding your patients and colleagues will rely on.

Finalizing Your Certification Plan

Every nurse practitioner chooses a population of focus, and your entire academic program has been designed to prepare you for that role. Upon graduation, you must demonstrate competence in your population by successfully completing a national certification exam, commonly referred to as the "Boards."

Each certifying body requires proof that you have completed your program, typically submitted by a faculty representative. For example, the American Nurses Credentialing Center (ANCC) requires an official form verifying program completion. Most schools will not send this form until the degree is officially conferred on your transcript, which can take several weeks. Check with your faculty early to clarify your program's submission timeline.

Reading and Using the Candidate Handbook

Every national NP exam publishes a candidate handbook. Think of it as your official guide; it outlines what you will be tested on, how the test is structured, and what to expect from registration through score release. Read it early and return to it often during your preparation.

Pay particular attention to the exam blueprint, which lists content domains and their weighting, and the reference bibliography, which identifies the textbooks and guidelines used to write exam questions. Align your study resources with these references. Review the testing policies for registration deadlines, rescheduling fees, identification requirements, and rules for remote versus test-center testing. Finally, note the candidate eligibility criteria, including documentation of degree completion and the timeframe allowed between graduation and testing.

This information is essential for avoiding errors or outdated materials. Many NP programs deliberately align their course textbooks with those listed in the handbook. Use that alignment to your advantage as you review for the exams.

When developing your study plan, map the content areas to your calendar in proportion to their blueprint weighting. Build a master list of key references and ensure you are studying from the correct editions. You can also tag your practice questions by blueprint domain so that your review mirrors the distribution of exam content.

About two weeks before your test, revisit the handbook to confirm all logistical details such as ID requirements, arrival time, allowed materials, and rescheduling policies. These details change occasionally and confirming them in advance helps prevent unnecessary stress on exam day.

If you require ADA accommodations or plan to test internationally, begin that process early. Documentation reviews and approvals can take several weeks.

Choosing a Review Course

Most graduates complete at least one comprehensive review course to prepare for the certification exam. The purpose is not only to refresh knowledge but also to refine test-taking strategies, strengthen clinical reasoning, and build confidence. Faculty often recommend using one review resource during clinical rotations to reinforce ongoing learning and another, more intensive review after graduation for final preparation.

When selecting a review course, look for one that follows the official exam blueprint, provides ample practice questions with rationales, and is taught by experienced NP educators. Flexible delivery formats such as live sessions, self-paced modules, or recorded webinars can help accommodate your study schedule. Courses that offer content updates as guidelines evolve are especially valuable.

Provider	Populations Covered	Format Options	Key Features
Barkley & Associates	FNP, AGPCNP, AGACNP, PMHNP, PNP	Live or recorded webinars, printed materials	Includes readiness testing; widely used in academia
Fitzgerald Health Education Associates	FNP, AGPCNP, AGACNP, PMHNP	Live, on-demand, and self-paced	Comprehensive pharmacology focus and long-standing reputation
APEA (Amelie Hollier)	FNP, AGPCNP, PMHNP	Video, audio, live, and question bank	Engaging instruction and detailed clinical reasoning
Maria Codina Leik Review	FNP, AGNP	Textbook, e-book, and app	Concise outline format with thousands of questions
BoardVitals	FNP, AGNP, PMHNP, WHNP	Online timed question bank	Adaptive review and detailed rationales
Roush Review	FNP, AGPCNP	Live and virtual formats	Strong clinical clarity and practical mnemonics

Provider	Populations Covered	Format Options	Key Features
Sarah Michelle NP Reviews	FNP, AGNP, PMHNP	Video modules and live crash courses	Focus on mindset and test-anxiety management
Hollier Review / My Amelie App	FNP, AGNP	Mobile app	On-the-go flashcards and short quizzes
PSI / ANCC Official Prep Resources	All ANCC exams	Practice tests and study bundles	Direct from ANCC's testing partner

Developing a Focused Study Plan

A well-organized study plan is your roadmap to certification success. It prevents last-minute cramming, structures your review time, and keeps your focus on the areas that need the most improvement. Your plan should be realistic, written, and flexible so that you can adjust as you progress.

Many graduates are tempted to revisit familiar material because it feels easier. A strong plan challenges that instinct by emphasizing weaker areas first, reinforcing foundational knowledge, and strengthening clinical reasoning through repetition and active learning.

1. Establish Your Baseline

Begin by taking a diagnostic readiness or predictor exam, such as the Barkley Readiness Exam or the APEA Predictor. These assessments highlight your strongest and weakest domains in assessment, diagnosis, management, and pharmacology. Use your results to identify content that requires targeted review. Most graduates find that physical assessment, neurology, and musculoskeletal systems benefit from extra attention because they depend heavily on clinical interpretation.

2. Create a Structured Study Schedule

Plan your preparation over several weeks, starting with the weakest systems and gradually reinforcing stronger ones. Integrate the 3 Ps so that each week blends knowledge and clinical reasoning.

Week	Focus Area	Key Activities
1	Diagnostic readiness exam	Identify weak areas and organize study priorities.
2	Neurology	Review differentials, CNS pharmacology, and red-flag findings.
3	Musculoskeletal	Reinforce injuries, autoimmune patterns, and imaging clues.
4	Cardiovascular	Study murmurs, lipid management, and EKG interpretation.
5–6	Respiratory & Endocrine	Review chronic disease guidelines and medication algorithms.
7	Gastrointestinal	Focus on common disorders, treatment steps, and screening intervals.
8	Dermatology & Final Review	Complete high-yield differentials and full-length simulation exam.

Set measurable goals for each week. Many students find that completing 50 to 75 practice questions weekly and reviewing all rationales, both correct and incorrect, improves comprehension and confidence.

3. Fine-Tune in the Final Weeks

In the four to six weeks before your exam, move from broad content review to focused test readiness skills. Follow a detailed calendar with specific daily tasks and complete full-length practice exams under timed conditions. Prioritize rest, nutrition, and physical activity to maintain stamina and recall.

During the final two weeks, avoid adding new material. Instead, repeat high-yield topics, strengthen weaker systems, and review the candidate handbook for testing logistics, identification requirements, and arrival procedures.

4. Track and Reflect

Maintain a brief record of your progress, noting what you studied, how many questions you completed, and your accuracy rate. Seeing your improvement over time builds confidence and helps you identify remaining weak areas.

Job-Seeking Strategies for Nurse Practitioners

The search for your first nurse practitioner position begins long before graduation. While most students begin applying during their final semester, early preparation makes the process smoother and less stressful. The strategies below will help you transition confidently from student to professional practice:

1. Begin Networking Early

Networking is the single most effective way to find your first nurse practitioner role. Many of the best positions are filled through referrals and professional connections rather than public job boards. Begin cultivating relationships as soon as you enter the program by:

- Building professional rapport with your preceptors, faculty, and clinical colleagues.

- Attending state or regional nurse practitioner conferences and local NP association meetings.

- Joining professional organizations such as the American Association of Nurse Practitioners (AANP), Sigma Theta Tau, or your state NP coalition.

- Maintaining an updated LinkedIn profile that reflects your clinical focus, certifications, and professional interests.

Be intentional about networking both in person and online. A simple thank-you message after a rotation, or a brief note to a speaker whose presentation inspired you, can lead to valuable professional relationships later.

2. Use Job Boards Strategically

Job boards such as Indeed, AANP Career Center, and PracticeLink can be helpful tools for understanding salary trends, regional demand, and position requirements. However, choose quality over quantity. Avoid applying indiscriminately to dozens of listings. Target roles that match your clinical specialty, align with your professional values, and fit your desired work-life balance.

Before applying, research the organization's patient population, practice setting, and mission. Reviewing online reviews and public quality data (for example, through CMS's Care Compare) can also give insight into an employer's culture and expectations.

3. Craft a Customized Cover Letter

Every job application deserves a personalized cover letter. Use this short document to demonstrate that you understand the organization's needs and can contribute meaningfully to its mission. A strong cover letter should:

- Reflect your knowledge of the organization's services and patient demographics.

- Highlight your alignment with its values and community goals.

- Provide a concise example of how your education, clinical experience, or approach to patient care supports their objectives.

Avoid generic phrasing or repeating your resume. Instead, let your cover letter show insight, curiosity, and enthusiasm. Employers often skim hundreds of applications, so authenticity and specificity make you stand out.

4. Prepare for the Post-Graduation Timeline

Expect a transition period of several months between graduation and your first day as an NP. This delay is entirely normal and reflects the multiple administrative steps required before practice can begin. These typically include:

- Graduation and transcript processing
- Completion of your national certification exam
- State licensure application and approval
- DEA registration (if prescribing controlled substances)
- Credentialing and insurance paneling with employers or payers

For example, a May graduate may not start work until late summer or early fall. Use this time to maintain study habits, attend professional development events, and continue networking. Staying engaged prevents knowledge gaps and helps you enter practice more confidently once paperwork is complete.

5. Prepare for Interviews and Professional Branding

Once you begin receiving interview invitations, treat each as a professional milestone. Review common nurse practitioner interview questions and practice articulating your approach to patient care, collaboration, and safety. Prepare brief stories that demonstrate critical thinking, communication, and leadership, because these illustrate your readiness better than memorized answers.

Update your professional wardrobe and ensure your digital footprint (LinkedIn, social media, email signature) aligns with your new professional identity. Employers frequently look up candidates online before or after interviews.

6. Evaluate Each Job Offer Carefully

When job offers arrive, evaluate them through a long-term lens rather than focusing solely on salary. Consider:

- Scope of practice and level of autonomy within the role
- Mentorship and orientation structure for new graduates

- Contract terms, including benefits, continuing education allowances, and restrictive covenants
- Practice culture, team dynamics, and patient load
- Geographic factors, such as commute time, community setting, and cost of living

If you are unsure how to interpret contract terms, seek guidance from a mentor, professional association, or healthcare employment attorney. Remember that your first NP position is a stepping stone, not a lifetime commitment. Choose a role that fosters learning, confidence, and sustainable growth.

7. Negotiate With Professionalism

New graduates often hesitate to negotiate, but professional negotiation is both expected and respected. Review salary data from sources such as the AANP National Compensation Report or your state NP association to understand market norms. Be prepared to discuss total compensation, including:

- Health and retirement benefits
- Paid time off and CME allowances
- Malpractice insurance coverage
- Expected patient volume and call requirements

Express appreciation for the offer while clearly outlining your priorities. Negotiation demonstrates confidence, preparation, and professional self-awareness, which are all traits of a competent clinician.

Faculty Tip

Your clinical skills matter, but professionalism and preparation matter just as much. Employers notice the candidates who are organized, confident, and easy to work with.

Accepting an NP Role and Leaving an RN Role

Graduating from your nurse practitioner program marks a major professional transition that moves you from bedside care into an advanced clinical leadership position. While exciting, this shift requires thoughtful planning to ensure a smooth and financially stable handoff between your RN and NP employment.

It's important to recognize that there will likely be a gap between graduation, certification, and the start of your first NP job. This period often lasts eight to twelve weeks, depending on how quickly you pass boards, obtain state licensure, and complete credentialing with your new employer. Planning ahead—both professionally and financially—helps minimize stress during this waiting period.

Understanding the Transition Gap

The shift from RN to NP does not happen overnight. Even after passing your certification exam, employers must verify your credentials, complete payer enrollment, and finalize credentialing paperwork before you can see patients independently.

According to the American Association of Nurse Practitioners (2023), administrative and regulatory processes are the most common causes of employment delays for new graduates.

For most new NPs, this means two to three months between finishing school and beginning practice.

Deciding When to Leave Your RN Position

Many graduates choose to remain in their RN role until certification or licensure is complete. Doing so provides income continuity and helps maintain clinical familiarity. Others prefer a short break to focus on studying or preparing for onboarding in their NP position.

Both options are valid; the best choice depends on your finances, confidence level, and employer flexibility.

Once you begin receiving offers, take time to evaluate each opportunity carefully. The terms of your first NP position will shape your early experience and professional growth.

Evaluating Job Offers

When reviewing your first NP offer, look beyond salary to the overall employment package. Important elements include:

- Structured orientation or mentorship support
- Defined productivity expectations and patient load
- Continuing education or CME reimbursement
- Coverage for licensure, DEA, and malpractice fees
- Clear prescriptive and collaborative parameters
- Realistic scheduling and work-life balance

Ask prospective employers how long credentialing usually takes and whether shadowing or observation is allowed during that period. Understanding these details helps set clear expectations.

Maintaining Clinical Momentum

Delaying entry into NP practice for more than six months can make it harder to sustain your advanced clinical reasoning. A 2021 *Journal for Nurse Practitioners* study found that new graduates who entered practice promptly reported greater confidence in diagnostic and prescribing skills than those who waited longer (Faraz, 2021).

If circumstances delay your start date, stay engaged through continuing education, certification review, or professional networking to keep your skills sharp.

Practical Transition Tips

To navigate this period smoothly:

- Set a realistic start date, allowing 60–90 days for credentialing.
- Communicate openly with both your future employer and current employer if working as an RN during the transition.
- Budget for at least two to three months of expenses.

- Keep your RN license active; it remains a prerequisite in most states.
- Celebrate the milestone. Your RN experience is the foundation of your NP expertise—both identities are integral to your professional growth.

Faculty Tip

As you transition from RN to NP, leave your RN role on good terms. Healthcare is a small world, and professionalism travels. The colleagues, managers, and mentors you part ways with today may become future references, collaborators, or advocates for your growth.

Key Elements of an NP Contract

Your first nurse practitioner employment contract is more than a job offer; it is a legal agreement that defines your professional boundaries, financial stability, and career flexibility. Understanding what should and should not be included protects both you and your employer while establishing the foundation for a healthy working relationship.

Below are the essential elements of a nurse practitioner contract, along with practical guidance for reviewing each:

1. Salary or Hourly Rate

Your contract should state your base pay clearly, whether it is expressed as an annual salary or an hourly rate. Be sure you understand how productivity is measured, since some employers use Relative Value Units (RVUs) or bonuses tied to patient volume or quality metrics. Ask how often you will be paid, whether annual cost-of-living or merit increases are included, and if productivity-based pay is realistic for your particular setting, especially if you are a new NP still building a patient panel.

2. Malpractice Coverage

Every employment contract should specify the type of malpractice coverage, also known as professional liability insurance, that is provided and who is responsible for paying for it. Two common forms exist. A claims-made policy covers you only while it is active. When you leave, you may need to purchase tail coverage to remain protected against future claims related to past work. An occurrence policy, on the other hand, covers any incident that happened while the policy was active, even if the claim is filed after you leave. This means no tail coverage is required.

Ask directly whether the employer pays for tail coverage when you separate from the organization, and confirm that the policy includes legal defense, board-complaint coverage, and your consent before any claim is settled. Verify whether the coverage applies to all professional activities such as teaching, consulting, or volunteer work, and request a copy of the policy for your records.

For a list of common professional liability insurance providers and coverage highlights, see Appendix G: *Common Professional Liability Insurance Providers for Nurse Practitioners*.

Below are questions to ask before signing:

- Is the policy claims-made or occurrence?

- What are the liability limits (common minimum is $1 million per claim and $3 million aggregate)?

- Who pays for tail coverage if I leave?

- Am I covered for volunteer, PRN, or teaching work?

- Does the policy include legal defense and board-complaint representation?

- Will I receive a copy of the policy and proof of coverage annually?

3. Continuing Education and Professional Development

Professional growth should be supported within your employment contract. Look for provisions that describe funding for continuing education (CE) and any paid CE days, as well as reimbursement for conferences, registration fees, and travel costs. Many employers also cover the expense of certification or license renewals. Employers who invest in your learning tend to value clinical quality and long-term retention.

4. Paid Time Off (PTO) and Sick Leave

Contracts should clearly outline the organization's leave policies, including vacation, sick leave, bereavement leave, and paid holidays. Confirm whether PTO is accrued throughout the year or granted annually, and whether unused time carries over or expires at the year's end. For part-time or newly hired NPs, clarify how time off is prorated to avoid confusion later.

5. Benefits Package

Your overall benefits package is as important as your salary. A comprehensive offer may include health, dental, and vision insurance, a retirement plan with employer match, and disability or life insurance. Some organizations also reimburse continuing education expenses, professional dues, and fees for licensure or certification. If you are entering a practice located in a rural or federally qualified health site, you may also be eligible for loan repayment programs. When comparing multiple job offers, look at the total compensation value, including benefits, not just the base pay.

6. On-Call Expectations

Be sure to clarify any on-call responsibilities and how they are compensated. Determine how often you will be on-call, whether duties are shared among providers, and if call involves only phone coverage or in-person visits. Find out whether on-call hours are compensated separately or included in your salary.

7. Termination Clauses

Your contract should specify how either party can end the agreement. Most contracts include both "without cause" and "for cause" provisions. A "without cause" clause allows either party to terminate the contract with written notice, usually with 30 to 90 days' notice, while "for cause" clauses outline specific reasons such as loss of licensure, misconduct, or breach of policy. If your contract includes repayment terms for sign-on bonuses or relocation stipends, ensure they are prorated so that you do not owe the full amount if you fulfill part of the agreement.

8. Non-Compete and Restrictive Covenants

Many NP contracts contain restrictive covenants, also called non-compete clauses, which limit where you can work after leaving an employer. Review the specific details carefully, including the radius, duration, and scope, since overly broad language can restrict your career mobility. If the terms feel unclear or excessive, ask for clarification or negotiate adjustments before signing. Even small changes in distance or duration can make a significant difference in maintaining professional flexibility.

9. Legal and Professional Review

Finally, always have your contract reviewed by a healthcare attorney or employment law specialist before signing. An experienced attorney can identify vague terms, restrictive clauses, or liability risks that could affect your career, income, or malpractice exposure.

Summary Checklist: NP Contract Review

Before signing, ensure your contract addresses the following:

- Salary and bonus structure
- Malpractice insurance details, including tail coverage
- Paid time off and CME funding
- Benefits and retirement plan
- On-call expectations
- Termination clauses and repayment terms
- Non-compete or restrictive covenants
- Legal review completed

A well-negotiated contract sets the tone for your professional success. Understanding each component protects your interests, enhances job satisfaction, and empowers you to enter practice with clarity and confidence.

Faculty Tip

Faculty see graduates sign contracts that limit their autonomy for years. If a clause feels confusing or too good to be true, have a healthcare attorney look at it. A short review now protects your income, your mobility, and your future practice choices.

Applying for State Licensure

After passing your national certification exam, your next official step is to apply for state licensure as an NP. This credential authorizes you to practice independently where permitted, prescribe medications, and bill for services within your population of focus.

Although certification verifies national competency, your state license grants the legal authority to practice. The process can feel tedious with its forms, verifications, and background checks, but it is an essential bridge between graduation and employment.

1. Maintain Your RN License

Your registered nurse (RN) license must remain active and unencumbered at all times. The NP license builds upon your RN license rather than replacing it. If your RN license lapses, you may become ineligible for NP licensure or practice.

Create a digital licensure binder with renewal dates, confirmation emails, and copies of both your RN and NP licenses. This organized record will save time when you later apply for credentialing or new positions.

2. Understanding the NP Compact

Unlike the RN Compact, there is currently no national NP Compact that allows multi-state practice. Each state has its own forms, fees, and requirements. You must apply for a separate NP license in every state where you plan to practice or provide telehealth services. Some states also require additional documentation for prescriptive authority or collaborative agreements.

The National Council of State Boards of Nursing (NCSBN) continues to develop a proposed NP Compact, but as of 2025, it is not yet active. Check ncsbn.org for updates if you anticipate multi-state practice.

3. Prepare Your Application Packet

Each state's Board of Nursing (BON) provides its own checklist, but most require:

- Proof of national certification
- Official transcripts sent directly from your university
- Verification of your active RN license
- Application form and processing fee
- Background check or fingerprinting
- Documentation of collaboration, if required
- Controlled substance education verification (in some states)

Download your state's application checklist before you test. Completing smaller items early, such as background checks or transcript requests, can significantly shorten your turnaround time once you pass your exam.

4. Plan for Your Timeline

Licensure processing times vary widely among states. Some boards complete applications within two to four weeks, while others may take up to twelve weeks or longer, especially in high-volume states such as California, New York, and New Jersey. Factors like background checks, prescriptive authority forms, and collaboration agreements can also affect how long the process takes.

To avoid unnecessary delays, contact your state board of nursing early to confirm its current processing times and submission requirements. Ask whether you can complete any components—such as fingerprinting or background checks—before receiving your official certification results. Submitting a complete and accurate application the first time is the best way to prevent hold-ups and start your NP role as soon as possible.

5. Tips to Avoid Delays

To avoid unnecessary delays in the licensure process, keep these key steps in mind:

- Submit your application as soon as you pass boards.

- Keep copies of every confirmation email, receipt, and submission.

- Ask your program faculty about typical state timelines.

- Follow up politely if delays occur, especially during peak graduation months.

- Do not resign from your RN position until your NP license is active or a guaranteed start date is confirmed.

Plan for at least 4 to 8 weeks of processing, and up to 12 weeks in high-volume states. Communicate your expected licensure date clearly to potential employers to demonstrate professionalism and realistic planning.

6. Maintain Your License Once Issued

Once your NP license is granted:

- Record the issue and expiration dates.

- Note the renewal cycle (usually every 2–3 years).

- Track continuing education requirements, including hours in pharmacology, ethics, or population health.

- Store both digital and printed copies of your licenses and CE certificates securely.

Set an annual credential check reminder to verify that your RN, NP, DEA, NPI, and malpractice insurance remain current. Regular updates prevent last-minute complications during renewals or job transitions.

Faculty Tip

If you are reading this and feeling overwhelmed, it's okay. There should always be someone in the office (with the potential employer) who helps you with this. Do you think physicians' figure this out alone? No! If there is lack of help, that should be a red flag. Also, stay calm and know this takes time. This is a long-term career move, not a RN job you are just picking up.

Credentialing

After earning national certification and obtaining your state NP license, the next step is credentialing. This process allows healthcare organizations, insurers, and hospitals to verify your qualifications before granting you the authority to practice, prescribe, and bill for services.

Credentialing confirms that your education, licenses, and professional record meet the standards required for patient safety and compliance. It can take several weeks or even months to complete, so understanding how it works will help you plan your transition to practice more effectively.

Employer or Organizational Credentialing

Hospitals, clinics, and health systems conduct internal credentialing to verify your qualifications and grant you clinical privileges. This process confirms your education, certification, active RN and NP licenses, malpractice coverage, and employment history.

The timeline varies depending on the size of the organization and the number of verification agencies involved. Smaller clinics may complete the process in a few weeks, while larger systems and hospitals often require more documentation and longer review periods.

Insurance Payer Credentialing

Insurance companies such as Medicare, Medicaid, and private insurers must also verify your credentials before you can bill for services. This step confirms your NPI number, DEA registration, malpractice coverage, and employment details.

Delays at this level are common and can postpone reimbursement. Begin payer credentialing as soon as your employer initiates the process and confirm whether the organization's credentialing department will handle enrollment for you.

Hospital Privileging

If your role involves inpatient or acute care, you must also obtain clinical privileges that define the procedures and responsibilities you are allowed to perform. This step is separate from state licensure and focuses on your scope of practice within that specific facility. Because hospital privileging meetings are often scheduled in advance, submit your paperwork early to avoid unnecessary delays.

Typical Credentialing Timelines

Credentialing often takes longer than new graduates expect. Even if all your paperwork is complete, final approval can take several weeks. The table below outlines average timeframes for each major type of credentialing.

Type	Who Conducts It	Average Timeline	Notes
Employer or Organizational	HR or Medical Staff Office	4–8 weeks (up to 12 weeks for hospitals)	Verify all documents are complete before submission and respond promptly to requests.
Insurance/ Payer	Medicare, Medicaid, or private insurers	8–12 weeks	Track completion by payer since delays can affect billing.

Hospital Privileging	Hospital Medical Staff Office or Board	8–16 weeks	Start early since committee reviews occur on scheduled dates.
Re-Credentialing	Employers, insurers, or hospitals	Every 2–3 years	Keep organized digital files for easy renewal.

Practical Tips for Smooth Credentialing

You can minimize credentialing delays and administrative frustration by following these practical guidelines:

- Keep digital copies of all licenses, certificates, and verification documents.

- Respond promptly to any credentialing or verification requests.

- Track renewal and expiration dates for all licenses and registrations.

- Communicate regularly with your employer's credentialing staff to confirm who manages payer enrollment.

- Be transparent about any changes to your name, address, or professional history to avoid delays.

Credentialing is often the single most underestimated delay between graduation and beginning to practice independently. Even with your license and certification complete, you cannot bill, prescribe, or see patients independently until credentialing is finalized. Begin early, stay organized, and maintain regular communication with your employer's credentialing team to ensure a smooth and timely transition.

Faculty Tip

Keep copies of everything. Everything. You will need to provide this information repeatedly. I keep both a hard copy and an electronic copy, organized by year and organization. Label files well.

National Provider Identifier (NPI)

The National Provider Identifier (NPI) is a unique 10-digit number assigned to every healthcare provider in the United States by the Centers for Medicare & Medicaid Services (CMS). It standardizes how providers are identified in all healthcare transactions, from billing to prescription writing, ensuring consistency across systems and payers.

The NPI was established under the Health Insurance Portability and Accountability Act (HIPAA) of 1996 to streamline electronic healthcare transactions and reduce administrative burden. Before its creation, providers used multiple identifiers issued by different payers, leading to billing errors and mismatched records. CMS finalized the NPI rule in 2004, and all covered entities were required to use it by May 23, 2007 (CMS, 2007).

The NPI serves several essential purposes within the healthcare system. It links every billable service to a single provider record, ensuring that all clinical and administrative data are accurately associated with the correct practitioner. This standardization allows for precise tracking of services, prescriptions, and reimbursements across multiple systems. By replacing the need for multiple payer-specific identifiers, the NPI also reduces duplication and confusion, promoting greater efficiency and consistency throughout the healthcare network. You can apply online for an NPI through the National Plan and Provider Enumeration System (NPPES). You will need your personal identification information, professional license and certification details, and your employer's business address.

Drug Enforcement Administration (DEA) Number

A Drug Enforcement Administration (DEA) registration number is a unique identifier issued by the U.S. Department of Justice that authorizes healthcare providers to prescribe, dispense, and manage controlled substances classified under Schedules II through V of the Controlled Substances Act of 1970. This registration helps ensure that controlled medications are prescribed and distributed responsibly, providing a framework for patient safety and regulatory oversight.

The DEA was established in 1973 through an executive order by President Richard Nixon, consolidating several federal drug control agencies into a single organization. The Controlled Substances Act, enacted in 1970, created a national system for regulating the manufacturing, distribution, and prescribing of medications with potential for abuse. As nurse practitioner roles expanded in the 1990s and 2000s, many states granted NPs the authority to apply for DEA registration, allowing them to provide more comprehensive care to patients.

Holding a DEA number allows an NP to prescribe and manage controlled substances within the limits of state and federal law. It also enables the DEA to monitor prescribing patterns for safety and compliance and is required for electronic prescribing of medications such as opioids, benzodiazepines, and certain stimulants.

Nurse practitioners apply for DEA registration through the DEA's official online portal. Applicants must have an active state NP license with prescriptive authority, a National Provider Identifier (NPI), and the physical address of their primary practice site, since each work location requires its own registration. In addition, all new applicants must complete an eight-hour federal training course on managing and prescribing controlled substances (Drug Enforcement Agency, 2025; Substance Abuse and Mental Health Services Administration [SAMHSA], 2023).

Some employers, particularly hospitals, government agencies, and nonprofit organizations, may cover or reimburse the cost of DEA registration as part of their employment package.

Collaborative Agreements

What Is a Collaborative Agreement?

A collaborative agreement is a formal written document that defines the working relationship between a nurse practitioner (NP) and a collaborating physician, or in some states, another advanced practice provider. The purpose is to outline how care is shared, ensure patient safety, and support professional accountability. A well-written agreement promotes partnership rather than hierarchy by establishing clear communication and shared responsibility for patient outcomes.

Although requirements vary by state, most collaborative agreements include several key elements:

- Provider identification: Names, license numbers, and areas of specialization for both parties.

- Scope of services: The types of clinical care the NP may provide under the agreement.

- Consultation procedures: How often patient charts will be reviewed and when collaboration or referral is required.

- Prescriptive authority: Whether the NP may prescribe controlled substances and under what parameters.

- Coverage plan: How patient care will be managed during absences or emergencies.

- Signatures and renewal details: Documentation of both parties' consent and the required review or renewal intervals.

A well-designed collaborative agreement establishes trust and ensures a compliant, patient-centered practice environment.

Why State Laws Matter

Your authority and independence as a nurse practitioner depend largely on the laws of the state where you practice. While your education, certification, and licensure establish your professional qualifications, your legal scope of practice—what you are authorized to do—is defined by your state's Nurse Practice Act and related regulations.

Because these laws vary widely, understanding your state's practice environment is essential not only for compliance but also for protecting your professional integrity. Many states still require formal collaboration, while others grant full autonomy. Knowing your state's framework helps you anticipate your level of independence, structure your employment agreements, and advocate for progress toward full practice authority.

To find your state's current regulations, visit the AANP State Practice Environment Map at (https://www.aanp.org/advocacy/state/state-practice-environment).

According to the AANP (2024), states fall into three levels of practice authority:

Practice Category	AANP Definition	Description
Full Practice	State practice and licensure laws permit NPs to evaluate patients, diagnose, order and interpret diagnostic tests, and initiate and manage treatments (including prescribing medications) under the sole authority of the state board of nursing.	NPs practice independently without required physician oversight.
Reduced Practice	State practice and licensure laws limit at least one element of NP practice and require a regulated collaborative agreement with another healthcare discipline or restrict the settings of certain practice elements.	NPs must maintain a collaborative agreement with a physician or other provider, often for prescribing authority or chart review.
Restricted Practice	State practice and licensure laws restrict at least one element of NP practice by requiring supervision,	NPs require ongoing supervision or approval from a physician to diagnose,

	delegation, or team management by another healthcare provider.	prescribe, or manage treatment.

How to Establish a Collaborative Agreement

To create a clear, compliant, and mutually supportive agreement, follow these key steps when establishing your collaborative arrangement:

1. **Review your state's requirements.** Begin with your Board of Nursing (BON) website, which typically provides official templates or guidance on acceptable language and documentation.

2. **Select an appropriate collaborator.** Choose a physician or advanced practice provider whose clinical background complements your own. For example, an FNP may partner with a family physician, while a PMHNP may collaborate with a psychiatrist.

3. **Clarify expectations early.** Discuss specific responsibilities, such as chart review frequency, consultation processes, and communication preferences. If compensation is involved, agree on terms before signing.

4. **Put everything in writing.** Avoid informal or verbal arrangements. Most states require a signed, dated agreement to be kept on file at your primary practice site.

5. **Review and update regularly.** Revisit your agreement at least once a year, or sooner if either provider changes employment, specialty, or location.

Chapter Summary

Beginning NP practice requires more than passing your courses or finishing clinical hours. Job seeking will start. Contract negotiation will occur. It involves a series of regulatory and administrative steps that determine when you can legally begin seeing patients, prescribing medications, and billing for your services. In this chapter, you explored the essential components of the transition from graduate student to practicing clinician, including national certification, state licensure, credentialing, and the identifiers that support safe and compliant practice.

You learned how to create a focused certification study plan by using the candidate handbook as your primary guide, aligning your study schedule with the exam blueprint, and selecting review resources that reinforce clinical readiness. Utilize the information on jobs, interviews, and contracts to be prepared. The chapter also walked through the application steps for state NP licensure, the importance of maintaining your RN license, and the typical processing timelines that vary across Boards of Nursing. You reviewed the purpose of organizational credentialing and payer enrollment, as well as how hospitals and clinics verify your education, training, competence, and legal standing before granting privileges.

The chapter further explained why every NP needs a National Provider Identifier (NPI) and when DEA registration becomes necessary for prescribing controlled substances. You also learned how collaborative agreements and state practice laws shape your day-to-day responsibilities and level of autonomy, emphasizing the importance of knowing your state's regulatory landscape before accepting a job.

Your goal is not simply to "get certified," but to move through each stage of the transition in an organized, well-planned way that supports a smooth entry into practice. Use the timelines and application checklists from this chapter to stay on track, then continue to Chapter 7 to learn how to build confidence, seek mentorship, and begin developing your long-term professional identity as a new nurse practitioner.

Chapter 7:
Thriving in Your New NP Career

Before you begin your first year as a practicing nurse practitioner, it is important to understand that professional growth does not end at graduation. It continues as you build confidence, develop clinical judgment, expand your professional identity, and deepen your leadership skills. This chapter is designed to help you navigate that early career period with intention, support, and a long-term vision for who you want to become as a clinician.

We will begin by exploring the transition from new graduate to practicing NP, including strategies for strengthening clinical confidence, understanding workforce trends, and using mentorship to accelerate your development. From there, you will learn how to incorporate lifelong learning into your professional routine, create annual CE plans, and stay current with evolving evidence and practice expectations. The chapter also introduces the foundations of NP leadership, showing how small daily actions, intentional communication, and advocacy help shape your influence within your team and the profession. A final section focuses on building a strong professional identity and planning for long-term financial stability so that your career grows in both purpose and sustainability.

By the end of this chapter, you will be able to:

- Understand the emotional and clinical transition from student to practicing NP

- Use mentorship intentionally to support decision-making, confidence, and early career growth

- Create a structured approach to continuing education and ongoing competency

- Identify opportunities for leadership in clinical, professional, and personal domains

- Build a strong and credible professional identity both in person and online

- Develop strategies for long-term financial wellness and retirement planning

The goal is not simply to continue working after graduation. The goal is to grow as a clinician, strengthen your professional voice, and build a career that reflects your values, talents, and long-term aspirations.

The Transition from New Grad to Professional

The transition from NP graduate to independent practitioner can feel intimidating. Many new graduates experience imposter syndrome, which is the persistent belief that their competence is inadequate even when their performance and preparation show they are ready. This experience is common among novice clinicians and is supported by research showing that new NPs frequently report decreased confidence and heightened uncertainty during the early transition period (Faraz, 2017). Faculty reassure students that confidence develops through repetition, reflection, and consistent mentorship.

Strengthening early practice begins with simple, intentional strategies:

- Create a structured "First 100 Days" plan with clear clinical goals and milestones.

- Seek constructive feedback from preceptors, collaborating physicians, and peers.

- Use AANP's Clinical Resources for NPs to reinforce evidence-based practice and stay current.

According to AANP (2024), more than 385,000 licensed nurse practitioners are practicing across the United States, with the workforce growing by roughly 9 percent each year. About 70 percent are certified in family practice, and nearly half work in outpatient settings. This expanding workforce reflects rising demand for NP-led care and increasing opportunities for specialization. The data below highlights the professional landscape you are entering.

Metric	Value
Licensed NPs in the United States	385,000+
Annual workforce growth	~9% per year
Primary care (FNP) specialization	70%
Median NP age	46 years
Practice settings	48% outpatient, 28% hospital, 10% academia, 14% other

The Power of Mentorship

Mentorship bridges the gap between education and independent practice. The transition from student to practicing nurse practitioner is one of the most formative and vulnerable stages of your career. The guidance of an experienced mentor can make a profound difference, offering clinical insight, emotional support, and a model for professionalism, integrity, and leadership.

According to the American Association of Nurse Practitioners (AANP), structured mentorship is one of the strongest predictors of long-term success for early- and mid-career NPs. The Fellows of the American Association of Nurse Practitioners (FAANP) Mentoring and Career Advancement Program provides a formal structure for growth, offering guidance in clinical mastery, leadership, academic advancement, and health policy engagement (AANP, 2024).

Formal and Informal Mentorship

Mentorship can take several forms, both valuable in different ways:

- Formal mentorship occurs through structured programs such as the FAANP Career Advancement Program. These programs pair new or mid-career NPs with experienced fellows who share similar interests or goals. The process usually includes defined objectives, timelines, and measurable outcomes.

- Informal mentorship develops naturally through professional relationships, networks, or shared interests. A colleague, supervisor, or faculty member may become an informal mentor simply by providing consistent advice, feedback, and encouragement.

What matters most is intentional engagement. Whether your mentor is assigned or self-selected, the relationship should be active, goal-driven, and built on mutual respect.

How to Identify and Engage a Mentor

A successful mentorship doesn't happen by chance. It's created through intentional effort. Consider these steps when seeking and developing a mentor relationship.

1. **Clarify Your Goals.** Define what you hope to gain from mentorship—clinical guidance, career advancement, leadership development, or strategies for balancing work and life.

2. **Seek Role Models You Admire.** Identify professionals who demonstrate the qualities you value most, such as strong communication, ethical practice, and community involvement.

3. **Begin Informally.** Start with small interactions such as asking for advice, following their professional work, or connecting at an AANP event.

4. **Ask Directly and Professionally.** When ready, make your request clear and respectful. For example, "I admire your leadership in women's health policy and would value your guidance as I explore advocacy roles. Would you be open to mentoring me for the next six months?" State your goals, preferred frequency of contact, and desired outcomes.

5. **Set Expectations Together.** Decide how and how often to meet and establish measurable milestones. Formal mentorship programs often recommend an initial three- to six-month commitment.

6. **Be an Active Participant.** Arrive prepared, complete agreed-upon tasks, and express appreciation for your mentor's time and feedback.

7. **Reassess and Evolve.** Review your progress every few months. If goals are met, transition into a collegial relationship; if not, refine your objectives.

What Faculty Recommend in a Mentor

Look for mentors who:

- Model professionalism and leadership.
- Provide constructive feedback and guidance during challenges.
- Encourage participation in AANP or state-level NP organizations.
- Uphold high ethical and accountability standards.
- Foster independence by helping you build your own professional voice.

Why Mentorship Matters

Research consistently shows that mentorship enhances both professional development and career satisfaction. Findings, as shown in the table below from the AANP Leadership and Mentorship Survey (2024), demonstrate that NPs with mentors experience higher confidence, career advancement, and retention.

Outcome	Without Mentorship	With Mentorship
Role confidence	54%	86%
Career advancement within 2 years	22%	63%
Job satisfaction	61%	90%
Retention after 3 years	68%	88%

Source: AANP Leadership and Mentorship Report (2024)

These results highlight that mentorship is not a luxury—it is an investment in professional longevity. Mentored NPs are more likely to remain in practice, grow in confidence, and assume leadership roles that strengthen the future of the profession.

Faculty Tip

The graduates who grow the fastest are the ones who actively seek mentorship, not the ones who assume it will happen naturally. A good mentor shortens your learning curve and strengthens your confidence.

Continuing Education and Lifelong Learning

Lifelong learning is the foundation of professional growth and clinical excellence in nurse practitioner practice. The American Association of Nurse Practitioners (AANP) emphasizes that maintaining certification, licensure, and clinical competency requires ongoing engagement with high-quality continuing education (CE). For NPs, learning extends beyond the classroom — it is both a professional responsibility and a personal commitment to staying current, safe, and effective in practice.

AANP data show that the average nurse practitioner completes 40 to 60 CE hours annually, exceeding most state renewal requirements. More than 250,000 NPs use AANP's CE Center each year to earn, document, and track CE activities. Approximately 37,000 students nationwide are enrolled in post-master's or Doctor of Nursing Practice (DNP) programs. Together, these numbers reflect a strong culture of academic growth and professional advancement among NPs (AANP, 2024).

Continuing education ensures that nurse practitioners remain grounded in evidence-based care while adapting to emerging clinical, technological, and policy changes. It also reinforces professional identity by cultivating lifelong curiosity, self-assessment, and accountability.

Creating a Yearly Professional Learning Plan

Faculty encourage NPs to view their CE plan as a personalized roadmap for growth — one that evolves with experience and aligns with both short- and long-term career goals. A well-rounded plan should include three core components:

1. **Required CE for Certification and Licensure Renewal:** Every state board and national certifying body (such as the AANP Certification Board or ANCC) specifies CE requirements, often including pharmacology and prescribing updates. Maintain accurate documentation of all completed activities, dates, and contact hours to simplify renewal.

2. **Clinical Competency and Specialty Advancement:** Select CE courses that strengthen your ability to care for your specific patient population. For example, a Family NP in primary care might focus on diabetes management, cardiovascular risk reduction, or women's health screening updates. Specialty-focused learning ensures immediate application of new knowledge to daily practice.

3. **Professional Growth and Leadership Development:** Go beyond clinical updates to study topics such as quality improvement, leadership, informatics, health equity, and preceptorship. These areas prepare you to take on new responsibilities, influence systems of care, and mentor the next generation of clinicians.

Where to Find High-Quality CE

The AANP CE Opportunities Portal offers hundreds of accredited, self-paced modules and live webinars across a wide range of topics. Many are available on demand, allowing busy clinicians to complete learning at their own pace. The platform features:

- **Topic variety:** Some examples include primary care, women's health, mental health, geriatrics, pharmacology, health policy, and more.

- **Conference content:** Access to recordings and materials from national and regional AANP conferences.

- **CE tracking tools:** Automatic documentation and verification of completed credits for AANP members.

In addition to AANP, state NP organizations, universities, and specialty associations (such as ACOG, ADA, or AACN) offer valuable CE opportunities. Attending live conferences or workshops not only fulfills CE requirements but also strengthens professional networks and collaboration.

Integrating Learning Into Practice

Education is most powerful when applied. After completing CE activities, take time to incorporate new knowledge into your practice by:

- Discussing takeaways with your team during staff meetings.

- Updating clinical protocols and workflows to align with current evidence.

- Implementing one new intervention or quality improvement idea each quarter.

- Reflecting in your professional journal or portfolio on how CE has influenced patient outcomes or your clinical confidence.

This ongoing cycle of learning, applying, and evaluating transforms CE from a regulatory requirement into a deliberate strategy for professional excellence.

The following table summarizes national trends in NP participation in continuing education and advanced learning activities, illustrating how professional development directly supports clinical excellence and leadership growth.

Learning Activity	Annual Participation	Application to Practice
CE completion	40–60 hours per NP	Maintains certification and clinical competency
AANP CE Center users	250,000+	Tracks, verifies, and stores CE credits
Post-master's or DNP enrollees	37,000 students	Expands leadership and scholarly roles
Professional leadership courses	Growing annually	Prepares NPs for management and advocacy roles

Leadership Development

Leadership in nursing is often misunderstood. Many nurse practitioners associate leadership with administration, management meetings, or politics, and instinctively avoid it. Faculty frequently hear new graduates say, "I didn't go back to school to be a boss; I just want to take care of patients."

Yet leadership is not a title, it is a behavior. Leadership shows up in how we advocate, mentor, teach, and innovate. The truth is that every NP is already leading in some way, whether or not they recognize it.

Why Many NPs Avoid Leadership

Several common barriers can make leadership feel inaccessible or intimidating:

- **Time constraints:** Clinical workload and productivity pressures can leave little room for professional growth.

- **Role confusion:** Some NPs equate leadership with management rather than influence.

- **Lack of confidence:** Imposter syndrome may lead new NPs to believe they are not yet qualified to guide others.

- **Negative experiences:** Past encounters with ineffective leadership may create hesitation or skepticism.

Faculty acknowledge these challenges but emphasize that small, consistent leadership actions can have a lasting impact. Leadership exists on a continuum, from influencing a single patient encounter to shaping healthcare policy at the national level.

Starting Small: Everyday Leadership in Practice

If the idea of being a leader feels daunting, begin with simple, intentional actions that demonstrate initiative and professionalism. Leadership often grows naturally from daily habits such as:

1. **Model professionalism.** Arrive prepared, communicate clearly, and treat every team member with respect. Consistent integrity earns quiet influence.

2. **Lead from the exam room.** Use evidence-based practice to guide care, share new research with colleagues, and encourage best practices.

3. **Volunteer for one small project.** Chair a safety subcommittee, organize a flu-vaccine drive, or present a short in-service to your team.

4. **Mentor and precept.** Offer guidance to students or new hires to strengthen both your teaching and leadership skills.

5. **Engage in professional organizations.** Join AANP or your state NP association. Even small roles, such as helping plan events, strengthen your network and visibility.

6. **Advocate in your community.** Write to legislators about healthcare access, volunteer at health fairs, or educate patients about preventive care.

7. **Speak up professionally.** Leadership requires courage. When you notice system gaps or inefficiencies, propose constructive solutions with professionalism and respect.

Formal Pathways for NP Leadership

For those ready to pursue formal leadership roles, AANP offers several structured opportunities. The Loretta Ford Visionary Leadership Program and AANP's Leadership and Mentorship initiatives provide mentorship, training, and networking for NPs interested in influencing healthcare systems or policy.

According to the AANP Leadership and Mentorship Survey (2024):

- 39% of NPs hold at least one formal leadership or administrative position.

- 75% of graduates from AANP leadership programs achieved promotion or expanded responsibility within two years.

- The most common leadership areas include clinic management (24%), academic education (21%), and professional organizations (14%).

Reframing Leadership for NPs

Leadership does not mean stepping away from clinical care; it means amplifying your influence. Faculty emphasize that leadership can be viewed through three interconnected lenses:

1. **Clinical Leadership:** Advocating for evidence-based practice, guiding care teams, and mentoring peers.

2. **Professional Leadership:** Serving in organizations, contributing to policy, and advancing the NP role.

3. **Personal Leadership:** Managing time effectively, setting goals, and maintaining resilience.

When viewed this way, leadership becomes less of an obligation and more of an opportunity to strengthen profession. Even modest contributions, such as teaching a workshop, writing an article, or joining a committee, add to the collective NP voice and expand your professional reach.

Faculty Tip

Many new NPs underestimate how much leadership they already practice. Leadership grows from small choices, not job titles. The clinicians who advance the fastest are the ones who take initiative, speak up respectfully, and contribute beyond their own exam room.

Building Professional Identity

Developing a strong professional identity is essential for long-term satisfaction, confidence, and credibility as a nurse practitioner. Faculty often ask new graduates a deceptively simple question: "What do you want to be known for?"

Professional identity is more than credentials. It is the integration of your values, behaviors, and reputation into a consistent and authentic professional presence. It influences how colleagues perceive you, how patients trust you, and how you advance within the NP community.

A well-formed professional identity does not happen by accident. It is built intentionally through self-reflection, consistency, and engagement with your profession.

Core Elements of Professional Identity

At the heart of every nurse practitioner's professional identity lies a clear set of values and a strong sense of integrity. These principles form the foundation of who you are as both a clinician and a colleague. Taking time to identify a few guiding values, such as compassion, accountability, or equity, helps clarify how you approach communication, documentation, leadership, and advocacy. When your daily actions reflect your core principles, your work naturally aligns with a sense of purpose and authenticity.

Professionalism is another essential element of building your professional identity. It is demonstrated not by titles or achievements but through consistent reliability, respectful communication, and ethical behavior. The way you respond to messages, manage conflict, or speak about others quietly builds your reputation over time. Each interaction contributes to how others perceive your credibility and character, and together these moments define your professional presence.

Equally important are clear boundaries supported by a strong ethical framework. Maintaining separation between personal and professional life helps preserve trust and credibility. Protecting patient privacy, avoiding emotional venting on social media, and exercising discretion in public or digital spaces all reinforce professionalism. Ethical boundaries are not restrictive; they are protective, allowing you to serve patients and colleagues with integrity while safeguarding your own well-being and reputation.

Together, values, professionalism, and ethics create the structure of a nurse practitioner's identity. They define how others experience your care and how you sustain confidence, credibility, and trust throughout your career.

Developing Your Professional Identity: Practical Steps

1. **Define Your Mission:** Write a one-sentence statement that reflects your professional purpose and values. For example: "I provide evidence-based, compassionate primary care that empowers patients to manage their health confidently."

2. **Shape Your Professional Brand:** Maintain a consistent and credible image across platforms such as LinkedIn and AANP Connect. Ensure your online presence reflects professionalism, warmth, and integrity.

3. **Engage in Your Professional Community:** Join AANP and your state NP association. Attend events, participate in discussions, and stay visible in your specialty to build meaningful connections.

4. **Seek Constructive Feedback:** Ask mentors or colleagues for honest input on your communication, leadership, and professionalism. Use feedback to guide intentional growth.

5. **Commit to Continuous Learning:** Stay current with emerging evidence, technology, and legislation. Share knowledge with peers or students to strengthen your expertise and credibility.

6. **Reflect and Realign:** Review your mission and professional goals annually. Ensure your actions and affiliations remain aligned with your evolving values and aspirations.

Cultivating a Professional Presence

A strong professional presence is built through consistency, respect, and intentionality. Faculty emphasize that professionalism begins the moment you engage with others, whether in person, by email, or online. First impressions matter, and the way you present yourself in those early interactions often shapes how colleagues and patients perceive your credibility.

Gratitude and humility also go a long way in strengthening relationships. Taking time to acknowledge the expertise of others fosters collaboration and mutual respect. These small gestures of appreciation create a sense of teamwork and shared purpose that benefits both professional and patient outcomes.

Reliability is another hallmark of professionalism. Meeting deadlines, responding promptly, and following through on commitments demonstrate integrity and dependability. People quickly learn that they can trust you, which builds confidence in your leadership and clinical judgment.

Finally, your online presence is an extension of your professional identity. Protect your reputation by avoiding unprofessional debates or negative commentary about colleagues, organizations, or patients. Maintaining discretion and professionalism in digital spaces ensures that your credibility remains intact and your reputation reflects the respect you show in your clinical practice.

Advocacy as Part of Professional Identity

The American Association of Nurse Practitioners (2025) identifies advocacy as a defining element of NP identity. Each practitioner contributes to improved health outcomes and access to care through their voice, visibility, and willingness to act.

Advocacy does not have to mean lobbying at the statehouse. It can be simple and local, such as:

- Educating a patient about preventive screening.
- Writing a letter of support for full practice authority.
- Joining a community health coalition.
- Speaking at a school or community event to inspire future nurses.

Every act of advocacy, whether large or small, strengthens both your professional identity and the collective strength of the NP profession.

Faculty Tip

The strongest professional identities are built quietly and deliberately. Your reputation forms long before you feel "ready." Show consistency, maintain boundaries, and treat every interaction as part of your public presence. People notice the way you carry yourself long before they notice your credentials.

Retirement and Long-Term Financial Planning

Why Financial Wellness Matters

While discussions about wellness often focus on mental and physical health, financial well-being is equally vital for long-term sustainability. Financial stress can quietly erode confidence, limit personal and professional choices, and contribute to burnout. Faculty emphasize that planning for financial security should begin early, ideally within your first year of practice.

A sound financial plan provides more than retirement savings; it offers peace of mind and stability throughout your career. Thoughtful financial planning allows you to make professional decisions based on purpose rather than pressure by reducing anxiety during job changes or life transitions. It also ensures that you have the flexibility to retire on your own terms.

Financial wellness is not only about preparing for the future but also about supporting your day-to-day sense of stability and confidence. Creating a clear, realistic strategy allows you to enjoy a long, purposeful career while maintaining the freedom to decide what comes next. In essence, strong financial planning strengthens both your professional longevity and your overall well-being.

Key Steps for Long-Term Financial Wellness

The following steps provide a practical framework for building financial security and supporting long-term professional sustainability throughout your nurse practitioner career.

1. **Build a Budget and Emergency Fund.** Track your income and expenses, especially during your transition from student to full-time provider. Aim to save enough to cover three to six months of essential expenses.

2. **Maximize Retirement Contributions Early.** Enroll in employer-sponsored plans such as a 401(k) or 403(b) as soon as you qualify and contribute enough to receive the full employer match. If self-employed, explore SEP IRAs or solo 401(k) options. Increase contributions gradually each year to take advantage of compound growth.

3. **Diversify Your Savings.** Supplement retirement accounts with additional investments, such as a Roth IRA, a health savings account (HSA), or a brokerage account. When possible, consult a financial advisor who understands the needs of healthcare professionals.

4. **Protect Your Income.** Safeguard your livelihood with disability and life insurance. Many nurse practitioners underestimate the financial impact of losing income due to illness or injury.

5. **Plan for Loan Repayment.** Develop a structured repayment plan for student loans. Explore programs like Public Service Loan

Forgiveness (PSLF) or state-based repayment options, especially if you work in underserved areas.

6. **Prepare for Career Transitions.** As your career evolves, consider future roles that align with your interests and energy level. Many experienced NPs transition into teaching, consulting, or part-time practice. Laying the groundwork early allows for a smoother and more fulfilling shift later.

7. **Create a Vision for Retirement.** Reflect on what retirement means to you with these questions:

    - Do you plan to fully retire or work part-time in a lower-stress role?

    - Once you retire, will you relocate, volunteer, or remain active in professional organizations?

    - Are you financially and emotionally prepared for this next phase of life?

Faculty Tip

Financial wellness does not happen by accident. The NPs who feel the most secure later in their careers are the ones who start planning early. Even small, consistent steps in your first few years of practice can compound into lifelong stability and freedom.

Chapter Summary

Growing as a nurse practitioner requires more than completing school or passing the Boards. It involves intentional development in the early years of practice, including mentorship, continuing education, leadership engagement, and the formation of a strong professional identity. In this chapter, you explored the emotional and professional realities of transitioning from student to clinician, including imposter syndrome, early decision-making, and the strategies that help new NPs build confidence through practice, reflection, and structured support.

You examined the importance of mentorship, both formal and informal, and learned how effective mentors accelerate clinical judgment, strengthen professional assurance, and improve long-term career satisfaction. Practical steps for identifying a mentor, establishing expectations, maintaining engagement, and evaluating progress helped clarify how to build relationships that support growth. National AANP data highlighted the measurable impact mentorship has on confidence, retention, and advancement.

The chapter also presented continuing education as an essential component of professional longevity. You learned how to create a yearly learning plan, choose high-quality CE offerings, and apply new knowledge to practice in meaningful ways. Leadership development was reframed as a behavior rather than a title, emphasizing that every NP influences patient care, team culture, and the broader profession through daily actions, advocacy, and involvement in professional organizations.

Finally, you explored the formation of a professional identity rooted in values, integrity, boundaries, and consistent professionalism—online and offline. Financial wellness was introduced as a key factor in long-term stability, supporting both career satisfaction and future planning.

Your goal is to grow with intention. The transition from new graduate to confident practitioner is a journey marked by mentorship, learning, leadership, and a clear sense of who you are as an NP.

Final Thoughts

If I could end on one final caution, it's about the debt/the money, the importance of clinical placement, and do not take jobs in desperation. You will have so many more choices if you start NP school debt free, learn to invest, and don't borrow excessive amounts to attend school. Just be very careful. Consult a financial advisor. Get into the weeds with your school about clinical sites. It is so hard to have enough for all. Be careful and selective as you build your experience and job portfolio.

I hope that you will seek me out in social media and join our private Facebook community, "NP Wisdom, The Parliament." I hope to share more with you in my legacy series.

Appendix A:
Self-Assessment: Exploring Advanced Nursing Paths

This worksheet is designed to help you explore which advanced nursing roles may align with your interests, strengths, and motivations. It is not a test, and it does not determine what you should do. It is simply a starting point for reflection.

Instructions: For each statement below, rate how strongly it describes you using this scale:

1. Not at all like me
2. Slightly like me
3. Somewhat like me
4. Mostly like me
5. Very much like me

Rating	Statement
	1. I want a career where I can diagnose, treat, and manage health conditions.
	2. I enjoy helping patients understand their health and make long-term changes.
	3. I am energized by direct clinical decision-making and critical thinking.
	4. I want the ability to prescribe medications and manage treatment plans.
	5. I like improving care by educating nurses and designing learning experiences.
	6. I enjoy developing others and watching their skills grow.
	7. I can see myself teaching in a classroom, skills lab, or clinical setting.

	8.	I like creating lesson plans, curriculum, or educational tools.
	9.	I am drawn to leadership, organization-wide decision-making, or operations.
	10.	I enjoy solving problems at a systems level rather than one patient at a time.
	11.	I am comfortable with responsibility, delegation, and complex coordination.
	12.	I like the idea of influencing policy, staffing, budgets, or quality outcomes.
	13.	I am fascinated by data, technology, or how electronic systems shape care.
	14.	I enjoy analyzing information to improve workflows or patient outcomes.
	15.	I like learning new software and teaching others how to use it.
	16.	I am interested in how health information is collected, stored, and used.
	17.	I am passionate about improving the health of whole communities or populations.
	18.	I'm drawn to prevention, public education, and addressing health disparities.
	19.	I like partnering with schools, nonprofits, or public health agencies.
	20.	I want to work outside the traditional hospital or clinic structure.
	21.	I enjoy reviewing details, policies, and documentation for accuracy.
	22.	I am interested in how healthcare connects with law, ethics, or regulation.

	23. I like writing reports, giving testimony, or consulting on complex cases.
	24. I can stay calm and objective in emotionally charged or legal situations.
	25. I want to support patients who have experienced trauma, violence, or assault.
	26. I am comfortable working with law enforcement or within legal processes.
	27. I can handle sensitive situations with compassion and professionalism.
	28. I am interested in evidence collection and trauma-informed care.
	29. I am curious by nature and like asking "why" and "how do we know?"
	30. I enjoy reading, analyzing, and applying research findings.
	31. I could see myself conducting studies, publishing, or presenting findings.
	32. I am patient, detail-oriented, and comfortable with long-term projects.
	33. I like coordinating services and helping patients navigate complex systems.
	34. I enjoy connecting people to resources and following them across care settings.
	35. I'm good at communication, organization, and long-term follow-up.
	36. I want to improve continuity, safety, and patient support over time.
	37. I want to influence laws, regulations, or healthcare policy.
	38. I enjoy advocacy, speaking up, and creating change at the systems level.

	39. I follow trends in public policy, healthcare reform, or nursing legislation.
	40. I want to use my voice beyond the bedside to shape how care is delivered.
	41. I see opportunities for new services, products, or solutions in healthcare.
	42. I like the idea of running my own business or independent practice.
	43. I am comfortable taking risks and thinking creatively.
	44. I enjoy the freedom of designing something of my own.
	45. I am calm and confident working with unstable or critically ill patients.
	46. I enjoy fast-paced environments like ICUs, ERs, or trauma care.
	47. I like procedures, complex monitoring, and rapid clinical decisions.
	48. I want to work with patients experiencing acute or life-threatening conditions.
	49. I am drawn to pregnancy, childbirth, reproductive health, or newborn care.
	50. I want to support birthing people and families throughout the perinatal period.
	51. I value holistic, family-centered, and lifespan reproductive care.
	52. I enjoy blending clinical expertise with education and emotional support.
	53. I am fascinated by anesthesia, sedation, and pain management.
	54. I like precision, focus, and responsibility in high-stakes settings.

	55. I enjoy working in ORs, procedural units, or surgical environments.
	56. I want a role with high technical skill and strong autonomy.

Scoring Guide: Add the ratings for each set of 4 statements:

Role	Your Score
Nurse Practitioner (Questions 1-4)	
Nurse Educator (Questions 5-8)	
Nurse Administrator/Executive (Questions 9-12)	
Informatics Nurse Specialist (Questions 13-16)	
Public/Community Health Nurse (Questions 17-20)	
Legal Nurse Consultant (Questions 21-24)	
Forensic Nurse (Questions 25-28)	
Nurse Researcher (Questions 29-32)	
Case Manager/Care Coordinator (Questions 33-36)	
Policy/Advocacy Nurse (Questions 37-40)	
Nurse Entrepreneur/Consultant (Questions 41-44)	
Acute Care/Critical Care APRN (Questions 45-48)	
Certified Nurse Midwife (Questions 49-52)	
Certified Registered Nurse Anesthetist (Questions 53-56)	

Interpretation: Refer to the APRN and non-APRN tables in Chapter 1 for a better understanding of these roles. Higher totals suggest stronger alignment with that path. This tool is not meant to give you a single "correct" answer but is meant to highlight patterns. Use this as a starting point for deeper research, shadowing, or career conversations.

- Scores of 16–20 = Strong alignment: Worth serious exploration
- Scores of 12–15 = Possible fit: Learn more before deciding
- Scores of 4–11 = Likely not a match, unless something else draws you in.

Appendix B:
NP School Interview Preparation Checklist

Research the Program

- ☐ Review the school's mission, values, and focus areas (primary care, leadership, rural health, etc.).

- ☐ Know which NP tracks are offered and why you selected yours (FNP, AGNP, PMHNP, etc.).

- ☐ Understand the delivery format (online, hybrid, or on-campus) and how it fits your learning style.

- ☐ Get familiar with the faculty. Know at least one instructor's clinical or research focus.

- ☐ Review admission requirements and deadlines so you can speak confidently about your readiness.

Reflect on Your "Why"

- ☐ Be able to explain why you want to become an NP in one clear, authentic sentence.

- ☐ Know why you chose this specific program.

- ☐ Describe how you have prepared academically, financially, and personally.

- ☐ Identify your strengths as a nurse and how they will support you in advanced practice.

Know the Role

- ☐ Review what NPs actually do in daily practice.
- ☐ Explore the different NP specialties and the populations they serve.
- ☐ Understand the difference between NP, Clinical Nurse Specialist (CNS), Certified Registered Nurse Anesthetist (CRNA), and Certified Nurse Midwife (CNM).
- ☐ Stay informed about the American Association of Nurse Practitioners (AANP) and current issues in the profession.

Practice Your Responses

- ☐ Prepare examples that show problem-solving, teamwork, leadership, and ethical judgment.
- ☐ Use the STAR method (Situation, Task, Action, Result) for behavioral questions.
- ☐ Rehearse your answers aloud with a mentor or peer until they sound confident and natural.

Prepare Your Materials

- ☐ Bring an updated resume and a clean copy of your personal statement.
- ☐ Confirm that transcripts and references were submitted.
- ☐ Keep a printed or digital copy of your full application in case specific details come up.

Demonstrate Professional Presence

- ☐ Dress professionally (business casual or higher).
- ☐ Arrive early or log in at least 10 minutes before a virtual interview.
- ☐ Silence your phone and close unnecessary tabs or apps.

Communicate Effectively

- ☐ Make eye contact and smile, connection matters as much as content.
- ☐ Listen fully and do not rush your answers.
- ☐ Keep responses concise, ideally 60–90 seconds.
- ☐ If a question is unclear, ask for clarification instead of guessing.

Be Prepared for Key Questions

- ☐ Why do you want to be an NP?
- ☐ What have you done to understand the NP role beyond internet research?
- ☐ How have you prepared for graduate-level academics?
- ☐ Tell us about a time you made a difficult clinical decision.
- ☐ How will you balance school, work, and family?
- ☐ What challenges do you see facing the NP profession?

Follow-Up and Reflect

- ☐ Send a short thank-you email within 24 hours.

- [ ] Reflect on how you felt about the program, not just how they evaluated you.

- [ ] Write down insights or questions while they're fresh.

- [ ] Continue building relationships with faculty and current students.

Appendix C:
Can I Afford It?

Follow these steps to create a budget projection. Be sure that you can afford it before you start.

Current Debt

- ☐ How much total debt do you have right now as a household?
    - o Personal
    - o Credit
    - o Car
    - o Loans
    - o Other

What Will NP School Cost?

- ☐ Cost of NP School
    - o Tuition & Fees
    - o Books, Technology, Supplies
    - o Clinical Site
        - Travel
        - Overnight Stay
    - o Clothes and Equipment

Income During NP School

- ☐ What is your projected income?
    - Work generated income year 1
    - Work generated income year 2
    - Work generated income year 3 (if applicable)
    - Projected student loan amounts:
        - Federal
        - Private

Projected Income AFTER NP School

- ☐ What is your projected income?
    - Work generated income year 1
    - Work generated income year 2
    - Work generated income year 3 (if applicable)
    - Projected student loan amounts:
        - Federal
        - Private

FINAL BUDGET

Now using the information above, create a budget for your NP school years. Then estimate payments after you complete school. Can you afford it?

Appendix D: Orientation Checklist

Bring these questions to orientation or your first advising meeting. They will help you clarify expectations, understand your program's structure, and build confidence before classes begin. After orientation, highlight any questions that remain unanswered and follow up within the first two weeks of classes.

Program Expectations

- ☐ What is the program's mission or focus (e.g., family, women's health, acute care)?
- ☐ Who is my assigned academic advisor or point of contact for program questions?
- ☐ What is the policy for leaves of absence, withdrawals, or incomplete grades?
- ☐ How do I access the student handbook and academic calendar?

Technology & Course Access

- ☐ What learning management system does the school use (Canvas, Blackboard, etc.)?
- ☐ What are the minimum computer and software requirements?
- ☐ Who do I contact for technical issues or login problems?
- ☐ How do I submit assignments and access feedback?

Communication & Support

- ☐ What is the preferred method for communicating with faculty (email, portal message, or office hours)?
- ☐ Are there writing or tutoring services available?
- ☐ Who assists with disability accommodations or counseling support?
- ☐ Are there orientation or mentorship programs for new students?

Clinical Preparation

- ☐ When do clinical placements begin?
- ☐ What is the process for securing clinical sites and preceptors?
- ☐ Are there placement coordinators or approved site lists?
- ☐ What documentation (immunizations, BLS, background check) is required before starting clinicals?

Financial & Administrative Questions

- ☐ When are tuition payments due each term?
- ☐ Are there scholarships, stipends, or tuition-reimbursement options?
- ☐ How do I access financial aid counseling?
- ☐ What are the deadlines for course registration and withdrawal?

Personal Organization

- ☐ How can I balance coursework with my current work schedule?

- ☐ What study and time-management resources are available?

- ☐ Is there a peer-support or cohort communication channel (e.g., GroupMe, Discord, Teams)?

Appendix E:
Study Tips for Pathophysiology, Pharmacology, and Physical Assessment

Pathophysiology Study Tips

Learning advanced pathophysiology requires more than memorizing terms. The goal is to understand the mechanisms of disease, which is how and why conditions develop, and to connect that knowledge to pharmacology and physical assessment. The strategies below can strengthen comprehension and support long-term retention:

1. Organize by system, not by lecture: Study one organ system at a time (e.g., cardiovascular, pulmonary). Create charts linking normal physiology, pathophysiologic change, clinical manifestation, and diagnostic findings.

2. Draw mechanisms: Use diagrams, flowcharts, or whiteboards to sketch processes such as RAAS activation or insulin resistance. Visual learning reinforces recall and deepens understanding.

3. Teach it out loud: Explain disease processes to peers, or even family members, in plain language. Teaching forces clarity and exposes gaps in knowledge.

4. Use clinical correlation: Connect textbook learning to cases. For example, after reviewing COPD pathophysiology, study a spirometry report or patient vignette.

5. Focus on patterns: Look for recurring physiologic themes such as inflammation, ischemia, or hormone imbalance. These patterns make memorization easier and support critical thinking.

6. Use active recall and spaced repetition: Quiz yourself with tools like Anki or Quizlet. Retrieval practice is far more effective than rereading notes.

7. Color-code and chunk information: Use colors to group related content (e.g., red for oxygenation, blue for perfusion). Break large topics into smaller sections to avoid overload.

8. Apply content to clinical scenarios: Ask yourself: What symptoms would I expect? What labs confirm this? This bridges classroom learning with clinical reasoning.

9. Reinforce learning with practice questions: After each study session, answer 5–10 review questions to strengthen recall and identify weak areas.

10. Preview before class and review after: Spend a few minutes skimming material before lecture, then review your notes immediately afterward to move information into long-term memory.

Pharmacology Study Tips

Pharmacology is one of the most demanding NP courses because it requires understanding not only the drug itself, but also how it interacts with body systems, disease states, and individual patient variables. These strategies help turn drug facts into clinical reasoning:

1. Learn drug classes before individual drugs: Group medications (e.g., beta-blockers, ACE inhibitors, SSRIs). Focus on shared mechanisms, side effects, contraindications, and therapeutic purposes. Once you understand the pattern, individual drugs become easier to learn.

2. Link drugs to physiology and pathophysiology: Ask yourself:

    - What part of the body does this drug affect?
    - Which receptor or enzyme does it target?
    - What disease process does it modify?

3. Use the "Big 5" framework for every drug or class:

    - Mechanism of action

- Primary use/indication
- Common side effects
- Major contraindications
- Key patient teaching or safety concerns

4. Master suffixes and prefixes: Drug name patterns often reveal class:

   - -pril = ACE inhibitors
   - -sartan = ARBs
   - -olol = beta-blockers
   - -statin = lipid-lowering agents
   - -azole = antifungals

5. Create mechanism maps: Draw quick flowcharts tracing how a drug works. For example, how beta-blockers reduce cardiac workload by blocking sympathetic stimulation.

6. Study side effects by body system: Organize adverse effects by system (GI, renal, neuro, hepatic) to recognize cross-reactions and safety issues.

7. Practice with clinical scenarios: Example: "A patient taking lisinopril develops a dry cough. What is an appropriate alternative?" These build board-style reasoning.

8. Use mnemonics strategically: Example: SLUDGE for cholinergic toxicity: Salivation, Lacrimation, Urination, Defecation, GI upset, Emesis.

9. Rely on repetition: Return to drug classes several times each week using spaced-repetition apps (e.g., Anki, Nursing.com, Quizlet).

10. Connect learning to real patients: If you are working as a nurse, look up the medications your patients receive. Real-world exposure makes pharmacology stick.

11. Check FDA updates regularly: Use Drugs@FDA for new approvals, warnings, and safety alerts. Staying current is part of professional practice.

12. Practice dosage and calculation problems: Even in graduate school, pharmacology requires math. Review conversions, titrations, and IV rates regularly.

13. Build a drug notebook: Create your own "mini-formulary" organized by system. Include class summaries, special considerations, and clinical notes.

14. Use reliable online tools:

    - EMPR.com – updates and calculators
    - Lexicomp – clinical pharmacology reference
    - UpToDate – interactions and treatment pathways
    - Epocrates – mobile reference and interaction checker

Physical Assessment Study Tips

Advanced physical assessment unites science, clinical skill, and patient interaction. These strategies help you move from memorizing steps to understanding what findings mean and how they guide diagnosis:

1. Review anatomy and physiology regularly: Revisit the relevant body system before each lab or practice session. For example, before a cardiovascular assessment, review cardiac anatomy, conduction pathways, and hemodynamics so that normal findings are clear before identifying abnormal ones.

2. Learn one system at a time: Divide your study plan by system (such as cardiovascular, respiratory, musculoskeletal) and focus on one or two areas per week to prevent overload and build confidence in exam sequence.

3. Use reliable visual and video resources: Tools such as Bates' Visual Guide or medical school YouTube channels allow you to watch, pause, and practice along with demonstrations of normal and abnormal findings.

4. Record yourself performing assessments: Video yourself completing a head-to-toe or focused exam to identify gaps in

flow, positioning, and communication, then compare to instructor demonstrations.

5. Practice on real people: Perform assessments on classmates, friends, or family members (with consent) of different ages and body types to improve adaptability and comfort with normal variation.

6. Master normal before abnormal: Spend time learning expected sounds, rhythms, ranges of motion, and appearance so abnormalities are immediately noticeable.

7. Create an assessment notebook: Include system-specific checklists, abnormal findings, clinical significance, and interpretation notes, such as "What does jugular vein distention suggest?" Use it in simulation and clinical settings.

8. Correlate findings with pathophysiology: When you observe an abnormal finding, ask yourself what structure or process is involved and why it is happening. This strengthens diagnostic reasoning.

9. Learn to cluster data: A single finding rarely forms a diagnosis. Practice linking related findings (such as shortness of breath + crackles + edema) to recognize common disease patterns.

10. Engage fully in simulation labs: Treat each session as a real patient encounter and request feedback on technique, communication, and documentation.

11. Become comfortable with exam tools: Practice using your stethoscope, otoscope, ophthalmoscope, reflex hammer, and penlight until handling them feels natural.

12. Document immediately after practice: Write or dictate a quick SOAP note as soon as you finish an assessment to build accuracy, recall, and habit. Include both pertinent positives and negatives.

13. Use mnemonics for exam flow: Examples include IPPA (Inspect, Palpate, Percuss, Auscultate) for most systems or OLDCARTS

(Onset, Location, Duration, Characteristics Aggravating/Relieving factors, Relief, Treatment, and Severity) for symptom analysis.

14. Learn the language of abnormal findings: Build vocabulary such as cyanotic, tympanitic, retraction, and egophony so documentation is precise and professional.

15. Partner with peers to alternate roles: Switching between examiner and "patient" reveals technique issues you may not notice from only one perspective.

16. Use validated assessment tools: Examples include the Ottawa Ankle Rules, Wells Score for DVT, or PHQ-9. These tools support evidence-based decision-making.

17. Reflect after each practice session: Ask yourself what went well, what needs improvement, and what feedback you received. Reflection accelerates skill development.

18. Apply faculty feedback immediately: Integrating corrections into your next practice session helps refine technique faster than passive review.

19. Use mobile clinical apps: Apps such as Bates' Pocket Guide, Epocrates Essentials, or VisualDx provide quick access to normal ranges, exam techniques, and clinical differentials.

20. Combine skill with patient connection: Physical assessment is both technical and relational. Explain what you are doing, protect privacy, and maintain empathy to build trust and confidence.

Appendix F
Clinical Toolkit

Clinical Bag Essentials

A well-stocked clinical bag reduces stress and signals professionalism. Preparation allows you to focus on patient care rather than logistics.

Category	Item	Purpose/Notes
Assessment Tools	Stethoscope	Invest in a reliable model you can use beyond graduation.
	Penlight	For pupillary and throat exams, carry spare batteries.
	Reflex hammer	Useful for basic neurologic checks; compact style recommended.
	Otoscope/Ophthalmoscope (if not provided)	Confirm site policy before purchasing.
Documentation Supplies	Small notebook or SOAP templates	For quick notes and case outlines.
	Pens, highlighters, pencils	Bring extras—writing tools vanish quickly.
	Reference apps (Epocrates, UpToDate, CDC Guidelines)	Use only site-approved devices and maintain HIPAA compliance.
Personal Essentials	Lab coat and student ID badge	Required in most clinical environments.

	Closed-toe supportive shoes	Prioritize comfort and safety.
	Water bottle and light snacks	Maintain energy during long shifts.
	Hair ties, lint roller, breath mints	Quick touch-ups for a professional appearance.

Capsule Wardrobe for Clinicals

Professional, consistent attire builds patient trust and saves decision-making energy on busy mornings.

Category	Item	Recommendations
Tops	3–4 neutral blouses or scrub tops	White, navy, gray, or black; breathable fabrics.
Layers	1–2 cardigans or light jackets	For temperature changes between rooms.
Bottoms	2–3 pairs of slacks or scrub pants	Wrinkle-resistant and comfortable.
Outerwear	Lab coat (with school logo if required)	Keep pressed; maintain a backup if possible.
Footwear	Closed-toe professional shoes	Non-slip, easy to clean.
Accessories	Simple watch with a second hand; minimal jewelry	Essential for timing vitals; avoid dangling pieces.
Quick Tips	—	Lay out clothes the night before; keep spare socks, deodorant, and a hair tie in your bag.

Meal Prep for Long Shifts

Sustained energy and hydration enhance clinical focus, emotional regulation, and professionalism.

Category	Items/Examples	Purpose/Notes
Main Meals	Grilled chicken wraps, quinoa bowls, bean salads	Balanced options that travel well.
Snacks	Nuts, fruit, yogurt, hummus with crackers	Maintain steady blood sugar.
Hydration	Refillable water bottle, tea bags, electrolyte packets	Prevent fatigue and headaches.
Containers and Tools	Leak-proof meal boxes, utensils, and napkins	Keeps food sanitary and organized.
Extras	Breath mints, hand sanitizer, small trash bag	Maintain hygiene in shared spaces.

Quick Strategies

- Batch-cook staples on weekends.
- Pack foods that stay safe without refrigeration for several hours.
- Keep snacks in your car or locker for emergencies.
- Hydrate throughout the day.

Appendix G
Common Professional Liability Insurance Providers for Nurse Practitioners

Insurance Provider	Coverage Highlights	Website
NSO (Nurse Service Organization)	One of the largest professional liability insurers for nurses and NPs; offers both individual and group policies; includes license defense, deposition representation, and consent-to-settle clause.	https://www.nso.com
Proliability (Administered by Mercer)	Offers malpractice insurance designed for healthcare professionals, including NPs; underwritten by Liberty Mutual; provides individual policies and optional business coverage for NP-owned practices.	https://www.proliability.com
CM&F Group	Established in 1919; specializes in advanced practice provider coverage; includes occurrence and claims-made policies, telehealth coverage, and flexible limits.	https://www.cmfgroup.com
Berxi (a Berkshire Hathaway Company)	Digital-first platform offering affordable, customizable professional liability policies; focuses on simplicity, transparency, and fast quotes.	https://www.berxi.com

Insurance Provider	Coverage Highlights	Website
HPSO (Healthcare Providers Service Organization)	Sister company to NSO; provides similar coverage for allied health and advanced practice providers; includes coverage for board investigations and depositions.	https://www.hpso.com
The Hartford	Offers malpractice and business insurance for healthcare professionals and NP-owned clinics; often chosen by those who own or operate independent practices.	https://www.thehartford.com
CM&F Group for AANP Members	Exclusive discounted rates for members of the American Association of Nurse Practitioners; includes occurrence-based policies and personal legal representation.	https://www.cmfgroup.com/aanp
Lockton Affinity Health	Offers customized professional liability coverage for nurse practitioners, educators, and healthcare business owners; includes optional business-owner coverage.	https://locktonaffinityhealth.com
Avant Healthcare Professionals Insurance (Regional)	Serves clinicians and healthcare staffing agencies; offers NP liability and license defense policies tailored for contract or travel work.	https://www.avanthealthcare.com

References

Accreditation Commission for Education in Nursing. (2024). *Accreditation*. https://www.acenursing.org

American Association of Colleges of Nursing. (2019). *Nursing faculty shortage fact sheet*. https://www.aacnnursing.org

American Association of Colleges of Nursing. (2021). *The essentials: Core competencies for professional nursing education*. https://www.aacnnursing.org/Essentials

American Association of Colleges of Nursing. (2023). *Graduate nursing program admission guidelines*. https://www.aacnnursing.org

American Association of Nurse Practitioners. (2024). *AANP clinical practice and education resources*. https://www.aanp.org

American Association of Nurse Practitioners. (2025). *About nurse practitioners*. https://www.aanp.org

American Medical Association. (2020). *AMA manual of style: A guide for authors and editors* (11th ed.). Oxford University Press.

American Psychological Association. (2020). *Publication manual of the American Psychological Association* (7th ed.). American Psychological Association.

Benner, P. (1984). *From novice to expert: Excellence and power in clinical nursing practice*. Addison-Wesley.

Commission on Collegiate Nursing Education. (2024). *Accreditation*. https://www.aacnnursing.org/CCNE

Drug Enforcement Administration. (2023). *Medication Access and Training Expansion (MATE) Act: New training requirement for DEA-registered practitioners*. U.S. Department of Justice. https://www.deadiversion.usdoj.gov/pubs/mate_act/index.html

Faraz, A. (2017). Novice nurse practitioner workforce transition and turnover intention in primary care. *Journal of the American Association of Nurse Practitioners, 29*(1), 26–34.

Faraz, A. (2021). Transition from RN to NP: Confidence, challenges, and strategies for success. *The Journal for Nurse Practitioners, 17*(10), 1228–1234. https://doi.org/10.1016/j.nurpra.2021.07.019

Harden, R. M., & Gleeson, F. A. (1979). Assessment of clinical competence using an objective structured clinical examination (OSCE). *Medical Education, 13*(1), 41–54.

Kesten, K. (2020, January 31). *In depth exploration of transition to practice NP residency/fellowship programs* [PowerPoint slides]. American Association of Colleges of Nursing. https://www.aacnnursing.org/Portals/0/PDFs/Conferences-Webinars/Presentations/2020/930_Kesten_Presentation.pdf

National Commission on Certification of Physician Assistants. (2024). *Pre-PA and program requirements.* https://www.nccpa.net

National Council of State Boards of Nursing. (2008). *Consensus model for APRN regulation: Licensure, accreditation, certification & education.* https://www.ncsbn.org

National League for Nursing. (2024). *Artificial intelligence in nursing education: Ethical and practical guidelines.* https://www.nln.org

NP Roundtable. (2019). *The Nurse Practitioner Roundtable position on post-licensure clinical training.* https://www.napnap.org/wp-content/uploads/NP-Roundtable-Position-on-Post-Licensure-Clinical-Training-2019.pdf

NPHub. (2025). *Preceptor placement and compensation data.* https://nphub.com

Nurse.org. (2025, May 14). *Nurse practitioner salaries by state (BLS 2024 Occupational Employment and Wage Statistics summarized).* https://nurse.org/resources/nurse-practitioner-salary/

O'Neal, M. B. (Host). (2023). *The DNP project podcast* [Audio podcast]. Buzzsprout. https://www.buzzsprout.com/1163231

O'Neal, M. B., & Stevenson, A. (2021). *The DNP project workbook: A step-by-step process for success.* Springer Publishing.

Parkhill, H. (2018). *Effectiveness of residency training programs for increasing confidence and competence among new graduate nurse practitioners* [Doctor of Nursing Practice project, The George Washington University]. Health Sciences Research Commons. https://hsrc.himmelfarb.gwu.edu/son_dnp/29

Substance Abuse and Mental Health Services Administration. (2023). *MATE Act training requirements and approved continuing education pathways.* U.S. Department of Health and Human Services. https://www.samhsa.gov/medication-assisted-treatment/mate-act

U.S. Preventive Services Task Force. (2023). *USPSTF clinical practice recommendations.* https://www.uspreventiveservicestaskforce.org

www.ingramcontent.com/pod-product-compliance
Lightning Source LLC
Chambersburg PA
CBHW051645230426
43669CB00013B/2453